VACCINES 2.0

VACCINES 2.0

THE CAREFUL PARENT'S GUIDE TO MAKING SAFE VACCINATION CHOICES FOR YOUR FAMILY

BY MARK BLAXILL AND DAN OLMSTED

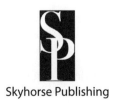

Skyhorse Publishing

Skyhorse Publishing books may be purchased in bulk at special discounts for sales promotion, corporate gifts, fund-raising, or educational purposes. Special editions can also be created to specifications. For details, contact the Special Sales Department, Skyhorse Publishing, 307 West 36th Street, 11th Floor, New York, NY 10018 or info@skyhorsepublishing.com.

Skyhorse® and Skyhorse Publishing® are registered trademarks of Skyhorse Publishing, Inc.®, a Delaware corporation.

Visit our website at www.skyhorsepublishing.com.

10 9 8 7 6 5 4 3 2 1

Library of Congress Cataloging-in-Publication Data is available on file.

Cover design by Qualcom
Cover photo: Thinkstock

Print ISBN: 978-1-62914-731-4
Ebook ISBN: 978-1-63220-171-3

Printed in the United States of America

Disclaimer: The information in this book is not intended to replace the medical advice from your doctor. The authors of this book are describing the various choices that are available. Mark Blaxill, Dan Olmsted, and Skyhorse Publishing cannot take the medical or legal responsibility of having the information contained within *Vaccines 2.0* considered as a prescription for any person. Every child is different and parents are encouraged to consult with doctors, therapists, and others to determine what is best for their child.

From Mark Blaxill:
To my beautiful daughters—Sydney and Michaela

From Dan Olmsted:
To my sisters, Rosie and Sally

CONTENTS

INTRODUCTION: YOU ARE NOT ALONE

January 11, 2014
From: "Concerned Father"

Greetings. My daughter London was born on New Year's Eve. As you can imagine I am incredibly excited. Unfortunately, I am also quite concerned as it relates to the potential dangers of vaccinations. My wife and I are trying to delay the process as much as possible until we feel that we are making a fully informed decision. However, our pediatrician and doctors are pressuring us and appear kind of annoyed when we attempt to query them on this topic. I was wondering if you know of a place we can visit (be it physically or online) that will guide us through this frightening ordeal without a vested interest.

God bless,

Anthony M.

"CONCERNED FATHER" IS NOT ALONE—and neither are you if you have questions and doubts about vaccinating your child. A recent poll found 9 out of 10 parents want more vaccine safety research as their top health priority; another reported 33 percent of parents believe vaccines do cause autism. More and more parents are foregoing or modifying all or part of the Centers for Disease Control and Prevention-recommended childhood-immunization schedule: A recent report from the American Academy of Arts & Sciences said 20 to 30 percent of parents selectively vaccinate, delay some vaccines, or have doubts.

With four million children born every year in the United States, that's a lot of parents in need of information they can trust about one of the most important decisions they will ever make on behalf of their children.

They're not getting it. Instead, blanket assurances of one-in-a-million vaccine reactions and "benefits outweighing risks"—the not-terribly re-assuring definition of a safe pharmaceutical product—are supposed to suffice. They don't.

What used to be a handful of "baby shots" for lethal illnesses like polio, smallpox, and diphtheria has ballooned in the past twenty-five years to vaccines for everything from hepatitis B on the day of birth to chicken pox at twelve months to human papillomavirus and meningococcal meningitis for older kids. So you'd think their safety had already been carefully studied.

But you'd be wrong. The big, booming safety claims you hear for vaccinations—separately and together, short and long-term, forever and ever, amen—are not supported by convincing evidence. In fact, when clear vaccine reactions occur in previously healthy kids, they are routinely suppressed or dismissed; even government officials ac-knowledge that only a small fraction are ever reported to the fed-eral vaccine-injury database. Parents, it's suggested, are either greedy and looking for lifetime compensation, "hysterical" and looking for someone to blame, or simply gullible and looking things up on the Internet that lead them to "confuse causation and correlation."

Vaccine-injury deniers act like concern about vaccination is a species of ignorance co-inhabited by UFO abductees and those who think Ebola is some kind of government plot. In doing so, they show contempt for the thousands of American families who have wit-nessed and tried to warn about what is truly going on. In a very real sense, they add insult to injury.

In truth, the chorus of concern about vaccine injury is much broader and deeper, and it can't be drowned out forever. A powerful, respected, and courageous voice for the truth was Dr. Bernadine Healy, former director of the National Institutes of Health. Before her death in 2011, Healy warned that the science supporting claims of vaccine safety was weak, and the willingness to investigate the truth was wanting.

Speaking specifically about autism, she told CBS News' Sharyl Attkisson in 2008: "I think public health officials have been too quick to dismiss the hypothesis as 'irrational,' without sufficient studies of causation . . . without studying the population that got sick. I have not seen major studies that focus on 300 kids who got autistic symptoms within a period of a few weeks of the vaccines."

In 2014, a senior CDC scientist named William W. Thompson confessed that data from a crucial study on the measles, mumps, and rubella vaccine had been improperly suppressed. The data suggested a link between autism and the MMR vaccine—specifically, that black males who got the MMR vaccine before thirty-six months had a higher rate of autism than those who got it later. He told Brian Hooker, a vaccine-safety advocate who secretly taped the call, that he was "ashamed" of his conduct and that of his colleagues. He went on: "Oh my God, I did not believe that we did what we did, but we did. It's all there. This is the lowest point in my career that I went along with that paper. I have great shame now when I meet families of kids with autism, because I have been part of the problem."

Thompson, who confirmed his concern about the study in his own written statement, was also recorded opposing a bulwark of the CDC-vaccination schedule—flu shots for every pregnant woman, whether the shot contains the mercury preservative thimerosal or not: "I can say confidently I do think thimerosal causes tics. So I don't know why they still give it to pregnant women. Like, that's the last person I would give mercury to. Thimerosal from vaccines causes tics. You start a campaign and make it your mantra.

"Do you think a pregnant mother would want to take a vaccine that they knew caused tics? Absolutely not. I would never give my wife a vaccine that I thought caused tics. I can say, tics are four times more prevalent in kids with autism. There is biological plausibility right now to say that thimerosal causes autism-like features."

These are stunning remarks by a CDC insider who has been deeply involved in vaccine-safety research for over a decade. If he has concerns about the timing, ingredients, and impact of vaccinations, so should you.

Even Dr. Thomas Frieden, the director of the CDC, which spends close to $5 billion a year buying vaccines for America's children and recommends the schedule of shots to states, has publicly acknowledged big gaps in our understanding of adverse events.

"In regard to growing vaccination resistance, what is needed is better data . . . to complete urgently needed studies of safer, more effective vaccines," Dr. Frieden said in a candid moment at the National Press Club in Washington in 2013.

Yet, when it comes to routine childhood vaccinations, federal officials have put the priority on wiping out infectious diseases of decreasing danger, not on eliminating vaccine side effects of increasing severity. Wiping out dissent is also high on their agenda. In 1984 in the Federal Register, the FDA made this revealing comment regarding the oral-polio vaccine: "Any possible doubts, whether or not well founded, about the safety of the vaccine cannot be allowed to exist in view of the need to assure that the vaccine will continue to be used to the maximum extent consistent with the nation's public health objectives." (The vaccine caused poliomyelitis in rare cases and was subsequently replaced by a safer version that didn't.)

In other words, it is all right to suppress the truth in the interest of getting everyone vaccinated. "There are groups out there that insist that vaccines are responsible for a variety of problems despite all scientific evidence to the contrary," then-Health and Human Services Secretary Kathleen Sebelius told *The Reader's Digest* in 2010. "We have reached out to media outlets to try to get them to not give the views of these people equal weight in their reporting to what science has shown and continues to show about the safety of vaccines."

But debate is never dangerous in a democracy, except to those with something to hide. As Healy put it: "First of all, I think the public's smarter than that. The public values vaccines. But more importantly, I don't think you should ever turn your back on any scientific hypothesis because you're afraid of what it might show."

One obvious study public health officials have turned their backs on: A comparison of total health outcomes between those fully vaccinated and those *never* vaccinated–the heart of the matter. "I think those kind of studies could be done and should be done," then-CDC Director Julie Gerberding said in 2005.

Gerberding left the CDC in 2009 after a controversial tenure. Only a year later (the minimum time required under revolving-door restrictions), she became president of the vaccine division of Merck, which produces more vaccines for the CDC than any other company. If you wondered why such studies haven't been done and probably won't be done, wonder no more.

This revolving door between public health and private profit— with our kids caught in the middle—ought to make journalists, pediatricians, and anyone else who is paying close attention highly suspicious. That it does not shows how a kind of vaccine orthodoxy, or even cult, has taken hold, in which vaccines are treated like "holy water," in the words of one critic, and the high priests of medicine and media excommunicate disbelievers.

Part I:
Why You Should Care

CHAPTER 1

THE STAKES
ARE HIGH

WE ARE NOT OPPOSED TO VACCINATION—only to current policies that have led to what we believe is the dangerously bloated vaccine schedule now in place. We don't reject vaccination entirely, although we respect those who do. But we don't think a tweak here and a tweak there is enough to tame the problems. And that puts us on a middle path between two camps. A fresh look at which vaccines kids really need and what risks they take when they get them—that's what this book is about. We hope that whether or not you decide to vaccinate, you will tread this path with us. We expect to take flak from both sides, but that's what seeking the truth sometimes entails.

The key question for America's health is not how to convince every parent to get every child every vaccine right on schedule; it is why, despite the general triumph of vaccination, so many children are so sick. We believe the epidemic of chronic disorders—from ADHD to asthma and food allergies to juvenile diabetes to, yes, autism—in this generation of children and young adults is related to the unchecked, unsafe rise of the current vaccine schedule over the same quarter century. The fact that one out of six American children has a developmental disability is not just better diagnoses; it's a brand new normal—and a nightmare. Disabled children struggle to learn, compete with the rest of the world, and have the independent and fulfilling lives that parents wish for their children.

This is the real health crisis America faces. But being in favor of a more cautious and open approach to vaccination is not the same as being anti-vaccine. "These triumphs of immunology are undisputed," wrote Harris Coulter about vaccines against illnesses like smallpox and polio. (Coulter's own work was instrumental in getting the government to adopt a safer version of the diphtheria-pertussis-tetanus shot.)

"However, as so often happens in human affairs, success led to excess. After taming these ancestral scourges, physicians sought new challenges and, in due course, directed their attention to the common diseases of childhood." Now the battle has shifted to chicken pox, measles, influenza, rotavirus, hepatitis—diseases that we would argue are either not worth fighting very hard or no threat to children in the developed world.

In too many cases we've traded "common diseases of childhood" for adverse events uncommon just a generation ago. These include acute illness, anaphylaxis, or reactions that can be fatal, as well as chronic disorders that range from asthma and juvenile diabetes to developmental problems like attention deficit disorders and autism.

Nor is it "just" children—many young adults now suffer from autoimmune conditions like lupus and rheumatoid arthritis. In a recent article in *The Atlantic* magazine, Leah Sottile, whose young husband has an inexplicable autoimmune disorder, wrote that in her close group of friends, "we know people with everything from tumors to chronic pain. Sometimes our conversations over beers on a Friday night turn to discussions of long-term care and miscommunication between doctors."

Nor is it "just" the United States—in a world of seven-plus billion, our country's population is more or less the "plus" to the right of the hyphen. Based on the confidence placed in vaccines in the United States, groups like the World Health Organization and the Gates Foundation, the world's largest charity, are charging ahead with vaccination programs in developing countries. There, such niceties as removing mercury from vaccines—as the United States started to do in 1999, albeit incompletely, and Great Britain did in 2004—are not observed, the better to spread the life-saving benefits of vaccination to the masses.

"Bill Gates: Vaccines Are Conquering the World," reported the Huffington Post on January 21, 2014, just ten days after Concerned Father sent his e-mail seeking a guide through "this frightening ordeal."

It is easy to feel alone. But it is nothing compared to the feeling parents have when they know a child's vaccine damage is real, and that no one will acknowledge it.

Anita Donnelly left this comment on our blog, AgeOfAutism.com:

> Once you get it, once you get that your toddler went catatonic because of vaccines, you are shocked and profoundly sad.
>
> Once you get that it didn't have to happen, that it was totally preventable, you add to the tragedy the knowledge that you and your child and all children have been brutally betrayed and violently poisoned. For money or for pride. By tragic hubris, or by cynical profit. But it didn't have to happen.
>
> And your child's suffering is for nothing. Your child's suffering did not keep some other child from getting chicken pox because they could have been protected without the participation of vulnerable children that they know how to detect [with proper testing]. No, your child's vaccine did no good to any child. And it prevented your child from getting full use of his destined life or her destined brain.
>
> Once all the little pieces click into place, it's like discovering a mate has been unfaithful, or a loved one has cancer, or that you are going to have to file for bankruptcy after all.
>
> It is something you simply cannot "unknow." And it hurts like hell to admit what has happened, how we've been lied to, and that our own lack of wanting to know hurt our infant.
>
> It is a betrayal beyond belief.

There's a broad consensus, one that includes most vaccine-safety advocates, that vaccination has important public health benefits. And there are culprits besides excessive vaccination to consider in the new wave of chronic conditions afflicting the United States and other developed countries. The Environmental Working Group in 2005 found an average of two hundred industrial chemicals in the umbilical cords of ten babies born in US hospitals. The toxic stew included "pesticides, consumer product ingredients, and wastes from burning coal, gasoline and garbage."

But in this crowded field of environmental suspects, vaccines stand out. They are widespread; their rise has matched the epidemics of inexplicable illnesses afflicting children and young people today. They are also highly invasive, injected directly into infants, bypassing the usual immune defenses and modulators—even reaching the fetus with toxic mercury and aluminum in flu and whooping cough shots now recommended for every pregnant woman.

But as evidence mounts that too many children are suffering serious and sometimes life-altering vaccine reactions, the medical establishment has simply doubled down, denying the frequency and severity of these problems.

Doctors, public health officials, and others will tell you "the science has spoken," that "study after study" refute any link between vaccines and serious disorders, that only "junk science" says otherwise, that whatever else may be triggering the rise in autism, it's not vaccinations.

It's sad to say, but that's propaganda masquerading as science. What you as a parent hear is more public relations and marketing than medical fact. That approach turns up regularly in shrill broadsides by pediatricians who can't be bothered to take a few minutes to hear parents out on their vaccine concerns—or read the troubling and contradictory medical literature for themselves.

"Pediatrician: Vaccinate Your Kids—Or Get Out of My Office," threatened a headline in *The Daily Beast*. "There are few questions I can think of that have been asked and answered more thoroughly than the one about the safety and effectiveness of vaccines," said a pediatrician who writes under the pseudonym Russell Sanders. He went on to assert:

> The measles-mumps-rubella vaccine does not cause autism. The HPV vaccine is safe. There is no threat to public health from thimerosal. I can say all of this without hesitation because these concerns have been investigated and found to be groundless. But no amount of data seems sufficient to convince people who hold contrary beliefs.

Don't trust him. The evidence for vaccine safety is nowhere near as clear as claimed. The studies *aren't* decisive. The "three p's"—pharmaceutical companies, public health officials, and pediatricians—have hopeless conflicts of interest that lead too many of them to dismiss your concerns and tell you to leave it to "the experts."

Don't buy it. Get all the facts. Make your own choice and make sure you find a doctor who will help you implement it. (We'll walk you through that in Part III.) Put your own child's welfare ahead of the "herd." Ultimately, the herd—our fellow human beings—will be healthier as more and more parents stand up for their own children.

That's why we say you are not alone. Concerns increasingly show up in pop culture—when *American Dad* says, "We really should have spaced out your vaccines" to his son Steve, who dreams of growing up to become a backup dancer, or when a TV detective says, "It's just like a vaccine but without the autism," as he injects an electrode under someone's wrist. Every joke, Freud said, contains an element of truth—a truth that, while not universally acknowledged, is increasingly recognized by independent researchers.

"A compelling amount of research suggests that children are getting too many vaccines, too closely spaced together, and too early in life," says Dr. Russell Blaylock, author of *The Blaylock Wellness Report*. "Vaccines for diseases that are of very little danger to otherwise healthy children, such as the chicken pox vaccine, tetanus vaccines, hepatitis B vaccine, etc., could be eliminated from the mandatory schedule."

Thousands of parents who have witnessed vaccine reactions are willing to attest to Blaylock's concern.

Over the past decade, as we've traveled the country, talked to countless families and met many children who have regressed into autism after vaccination, we've heard the same story countless times. True, each one is different in terms of exact timing, symptoms, and outcomes, but the pattern in these repeated accounts is clear. They are not "mere anecdotes," not simply the testimony of angry, anxious, or "hysterical" moms looking for someone to blame or sue.

The American Academy of Pediatrics refers those with such concerns to the National Network for Immunization Information, which it helps fund. Under "Vaccine Safety: Cause or Coincidence," the NNII (immunizationinfo.org) states:

> Many vaccines are given to children at the ages when developmental and other problems are being recognized for the

first time. Because something happened at about the same time that a vaccine was given does not mean that the vaccine caused the problem.

Tell that to Abdulkadir Khalif, an African immigrant to Minneapolis, who wrote on our blog:

> I have a gut feeling (trust your gut feelings always) that my son was affected by what got into his body around the time he was 18 months. My son grew up a normal, healthy and bouncing baby. He started speaking a few words by the time he was about 15 months. He waited for me at the door every-day as I got back home from work and welcomed me inside.
>
> He knew how I opened the door and the approximate time I came home each day. He raced down the stairs and hugged me, then held my hand and led me inside. I looked forward to those moments and they were perfect moments as they relieved me of the day's tensions and small workplace frustrations. Then one day, I came home and he did not welcome me as was his wont.
>
> A few days earlier, Abdimalik got his 18 months MMR vaccine as scheduled. I still remember that day. His mother was coming back from his appointment and passed my place of work to give me a ride home. Abdimalik was sitting in his car seat, very quiet, subdued and absent minded. As I took my seat I glanced back wondering if he was asleep or not. He was seated squarely in his seat but was looking straight ahead at a point in space. I called out to him and he did not respond. I shook him and he did not move. I looked at my wife and asked what happened and she explained where they came from and that everything went well. She explained how he thanked the nurse as she put a sticker on his chest before the injection in order to build rapport. After that we rode home in silence and life was never the same again.
>
> On all subsequent days after that, Abdimalik went from one extreme behavioural problem to another. Fortunately he did not have seizures or vomiting like many other kids

we came to know. But he manifested all other behaviours like tantrums, biting, sleeplessness etc. We spent the entire next winter virtually awake at nights, relieving each other and trying everything possible to calm him down and put him to sleep. The doctors we visited knew exactly what the problem was but dare not tell us. One of them finally referred us to the school district, and there we heard the word "autism" for the first time.

As you ponder vaccine decisions, it's also worth looking at www.followingvaccinations.com, a site that collects simple, stark accounts of vaccine injury. Among the more than two thousand responses— and counting—collected by founder Joan Campbell:

Stephanie A.   At age 4, I had the DTaP, I remember my leg doubled in size. My mom said the Dr said I was allergic to the pertussis. She said my personality changed I started to wet the bed and was never the same. Now, 35 I have had over a dozen surgeries for Crohn's colitis.

Valerie A.   My son had adverse reactions to all of his shots and after effects from them like eczema, hives, etc. His doctor never reported any of them even when he was hospitalized a few days after the shots because his fever wouldn't go below 104 for days. Doctors usually don't-so the stats that the doctors give you on their information sheets and the number put out there by the CDC and AAP are WAY off!

Gavin B. was born June 26, 2003. Like any parent who thinks they are doing the right thing he was vaxxed on CDC schedule. I had zero education about vaccines. Only the paper his doctors gave me seconds before he was jabbed. 17.5 hrs from his 4 mo boosters he died. Immediately from the shots his fever soared, he became lethargic and lost his appetite. The nurse from the office told me his reaction was normal and to give him Tylenol and let him sleep. I could not wake him and rushed him to the hospital in what seemed to be the longest

5 minutes of my life. After hrs of tubes and more injections and air pumps he was pronounced dead. The ME said it was SIDS. I asked him if it could be related to the vaccines because he was so healthy till then. He told me the vaccines are safe that it couldn't be from them. That SIDS just happens with no explanation. I love him more than anything. Everyone loves him more than anything.

Once again, it is easy to feel alone—especially, as is clear from these accounts, when doctors are reluctant to report or even recognize adverse events. Yet more and more studies link vaccination and a wide range of injuries. Ginger Taylor, the mother of a child diagnosed with autism, and an activist for safer vaccines, has compiled a list of eighty-eight published, peer-reviewed scientific papers that point to a possible relationship between autism and vaccines.

Catherine DeSoto, a professor at the University of Northern Iowa, conducted an elegantly simple search of the database of peer-reviewed medical papers, PubMed, and found that studies that linked vaccine mercury and autism outweighed those that didn't.

Meanwhile, two scientists cast their nets worldwide and came back with evidence linking vaccination in the first year of life to infant death. The trend was counterintuitive but consistent: "*Nations that require more vaccine doses tend to have higher infant mortality rates.*" [emphasis in original]

"The infant mortality rate (IMR) is one of the most important measures of child health and overall development in countries," authors Miller and Goldman reported in the 2011 study. "The US childhood immunization schedule requires 26 vaccine doses for infants aged less than 1 year, the most in the world, yet 33 nations have better IMRs."

"All nations—rich and poor, advanced and developing—have an obligation to determine whether their immunization schedules are achieving their desired goals."

As do all of us.

You are not alone, because even Congress is pressing for answers. At a hearing before a congressional oversight committee in November

2012, representatives from both sides of the aisle raised the same questions parents have been asking for years.

"I've had so many parents write to me or come to me saying they had a healthy child who then got ten, nine, six vaccines at one time [and] that child changed overnight," said Rep. Carolyn Maloney, Democrat, of New York. "Why does the schedule require a child to receive so many vaccines in such a short period? I'm totally for [vaccines] but why do you have to cram nine, or six, at a time when the verbal evidence seems so strong from so many people?"

"I'm just sitting and I'm listening to all this," said Rep. Elijah Cummings, Democrat, of Maryland and the ranking minority member. "There's something wrong with this picture. . . . When you've got this combination of shots and you go from one in 10,000 to one in 88 [the autism rate increase in two decades], it seems to me that somebody would say, let's put the brakes on this. And at least, let's try to figure out whether, if I'm giving a baby nine shots in a day . . . how much impact that's having. I mean, if they gave me nine shots. . . . [Addressing government witnesses:] I wish you could see the people behind you. There are grown men that have been crying behind you, and women—crying. Let's err on the side of keeping children safe. Even if we have to do a pause and give children one shot a day."

The committee chair, Darrell Issa, Republican of California, pushed the government witnesses as well. "Was there autism before there was vaccination?" Issa asked. The witnesses claimed there was, but once again the evidence is the opposite: the first autism cases were reported among children born in the 1930s, when organic mercury was first used in vaccines. Family backgrounds link them to the toxic chemical.

If members of Congress can ask these questions of CDC and National Institutes of Health officials, you should feel empowered to ask them of your own health care providers and to demand that the answers make sense to you and for you and *your* child.

The irony, we believe, is this: Congress itself triggered the crisis that has led to the need for a critical new look at the immunization schedule—for *Vaccines 2.0*. First, we need to pause for a moment, turn back the clock, and explain how it came to this.

CHAPTER 2

THEY'RE EXPERIMENTING ON YOUR CHILDREN

WELCOME TO THE UNITED STATES IN THE YEAR 1986. President Ronald Reagan is in his second term, the economy is booming after a deep manufacturing recession, and the Oprah Winfrey show is hitting national television. In January, the Challenger explodes. Radio Shack advertises the new disk-based Tandy 600: "With telecom and the Tandy 600's built-in modem, you're able to communicate with other computers over phone lines." Life was different, but not radically so.

If you were born in 1986, your parents took you to the doctor at two months of age for your first well-baby visit. At that visit, you got your first vaccines—the polio vaccine (three more would follow by age six) and the combined diphtheria-pertussis-tetanus shot or DPT (four more by age six). At fifteen months, you'd get the combination mumps-measles-rubella shot, or MMR.

And that was that. Seven vaccines— including the three individual components of the combination MMR and DPT shots—by the time you entered school, given in a total of ten shots; none before two months; and no more than two inoculations per visit.

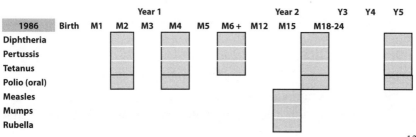

In general in 1986, America's children were growing up healthy and happy. No one was talking about a plague of infectious disease, except for AIDS. No one was talking about autism, either: The autism rate was 1 in 1,500, not much more than it was when it was first observed in the medical literature in the 1940s. Asthma was rare. The infant mortality rate was 10.4 per 1,000 live births, down almost fourfold from 38.3 at the end of World War II thanks to the rise of antibiotics, better food safety standards, and efforts to clean up the environment. It was one of the lowest rates of infant deaths in the world.

Now welcome to America today. Barack Obama is in his second term. The economy is nearly back on track after the financial crash of 2008. Radio Shack runs a Super Bowl ad poking fun at itself: "The '80s called, they want their store back."

But when it comes to vaccinations, things *are* radically different. If you were a New Year's baby like Concerned Father's, you were exposed to your first vaccines while still in the womb—a Tdap shot and the influenza vaccine recommended by the CDC for all pregnant women. In many cases, the influenza shot contains mercury, a high percentage of which ends up in the developing fetus as the mother's body tries to excrete it.

Within hours of birth, you'd receive the vaccination against hepatitis B, a disease most common in IV drug users and people with multiple sex partners, followed in coming months by two more.

At two months, you'd get a shot against rotavirus, with two more to follow; the DTaP shot, with four more to come; the Hib vaccine; the pneumococcal shot; and the polio vaccine, all with three more to come.

But wait, there's more. After that first flu shot in the womb, you'd get them annually, starting at 6 months (the first time twice, separated by a month); plus an MMR shot at 12–15 months, with a booster at 4–6 years; plus a chicken pox shot at 12–15 months, also with a booster at 4–6 years; plus two hepatitis A shots beginning as early as 12 months. And you'd get all of this by the age of 6.

So a typical child entering kindergarten would have gotten fourteen vaccines, double the number in 1986, in a total of forty-nine injections—almost five times as many. Most of them come within the first year of life. At six months, a baby routinely faces a real traffic jam: nine vaccines in seven shots—DTaP, polio, hepatitis B, Hib, pneumococcal, polio, and influenza.

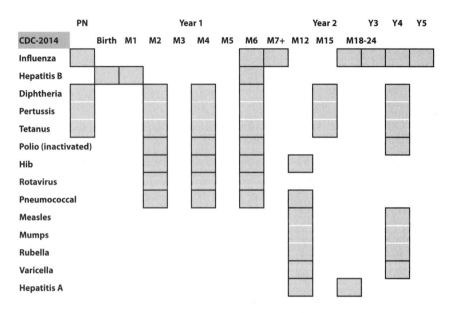

Then come a Tdap shot at age 11–12, three human papillomavirus vaccines at age 11–12, and two meningococcal vaccines at 11–12 and 16.

Why, you might ask, is this a problem? Isn't this the march of medical progress, and shouldn't we all just stand and gratefully salute as it passes by?

The problem is threefold. First, more medicine—like more food—isn't necessarily a good thing, especially when it is given for something that hasn't happened, might not happen, and might not be serious if it did happen. Injecting healthy infants with increasing numbers of man-made substances at very early stages in development is inherently risky, especially when the people most certain to benefit are those who get paid to make and promote these products.

When those individuals have power and a platform, they can push the whole system out of balance.

In broad terms, Americans seem to understand this. As a father of two said to us: "We all believe there are cases of over-doctoring—antibiotics, end of life care, and so on." News reports echo that common view every day. "Too many Americans are taking way too many antibiotics every year," Diane Sawyer said on ABC World News Tonight in October 2012. She didn't need to cite her sources, since everyone in the medical community agrees (though they often blame demanding patients). Overuse of medication for attention disorders in children is the stuff of *New York Times* front-page investigations. Cutting down on needless medical procedures is a prime goal of health-care reform.

So, contrary to Mac West, too much of a good thing is not necessarily wonderful. Second, the companies that produce these "good things"—global pharmaceutical giants—do not have a record of being your best friend. In the case of Vioxx, Merck allegedly softened study results to obscure the fact it was causing thousands of heart attacks and strokes, then fought every court case until settling for $6 billion (and promoting the lawyer who devised the strategy to president of the company, while hiring Julie Gerberding, former director of the CDC, to run its vaccine division). It also created a fake medical journal in Australia and filled it with friendly "research."

In 2013, Johnson & Johnson paid $2.2 billion in criminal and civil fines for peddling the antipsychotic drug Risperdal to people for whom it was not intended. In 2014, a subsidiary of GlaxoSmithKline was found guilty of charges and fined half a billion dollars in China for bribing doctors and officials. (Glaxo recently made news when it decided to *stop* paying doctors to promote its drugs, a practice most people were probably appalled to learn happened in the first place.)

Eli Lilly paid more than a billion dollars to thousands of patients who said they developed diabetes and other problems after taking its antipsychotic drug, Zyprexa.

This catalog of corporate horrors extends to drug makers' vaccine divisions. Why would it not?

In 2008, we obtained an inter-office memorandum from 1979 about distribution of Wyeth's DPT vaccine. A series of sudden-infant deaths in Tennessee prompted Wyeth officials to make sure entire lots of vials were no longer distributed in the same place. "After the reporting of the SID cases in Tennessee," the memo says, "we discussed the merits of limiting distribution of a large number of vials to a single state, county or city health department and obtained agreement from the senior management staff to proceed with such a plan."

There could be only one reason: To avoid detection of "hot lots," batches of vaccines that trigger unusually frequent or severe adverse events, like SIDS. Burying evidence of hot lots might benefit Wyeth, but it could lead to more deaths or illnesses that were not correctly diagnosed or properly medically treated.

The beat goes on. In 2012, two former Merck scientists filed a whistleblower suit, claiming the company traded children's health to protect monopoly profits and engaged in a systematic, elaborate, and ongoing fraud to do so. The alleged fraud: a multi-year effort to hide the fact that the mumps vaccine is no longer anywhere near as effective as Merck claims. In 2014 a federal judge refused to dismiss the claim. Vaccine manufacturers often act as though they are above the law. That's because in a very real sense, they are.

Which brings us back to 1986, when everything changed. That year, Merck brought in about $140 million from its vaccine business, primarily from the MMR II combination vaccine. Overall, total vaccine-industry revenues worldwide were around half a billion dollars. That sounds like a lot—but stand back.

By 2013, Merck's vaccine business was hauling in nearly forty times as much as in 1986—$5.156 *billion* for the MMR II; ProQuad® (the MMR plus chicken pox); Varivax, the single chicken pox shot; the Gardasil® vaccine against the human papillomavirus; the Recombivax B® hepatitis B vaccine; RotaTeqV vaccine against rotavirus; and Pneumovax® against pneumococcal meningitis, among other vaccines.

Vaccines became a blockbuster business for the top pharma companies after NCVIA

Revenues by company: 1985-2013

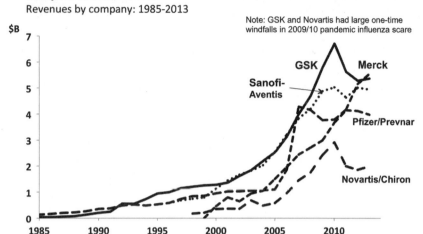

Note: GSK and Novartis had large one-time windfalls in 2009/10 pandemic influenza scare

Sources: Merck revenues provided directly in 1987-2013 Annual Reports. GSK revenue history from annual reports of GSK 2000-2013, SmithKline Beecham 1990-2000 and SmithKline Beckman press releases; Sanofi-Aventis revenues history from annual reports of Sanofi-Aventis 2004-2013, Aventis 2001-2002, Rhone Poulenc 1997 press release; Pfizer revenue is Prevnar only, and from Wyeth and Pfizer annual reports; Novartis revenue is from Chiron annual reports until 2006 acquisition by Novartis

By 2013, the total vaccine industry was taking in $24 billion a year from vaccines, up from less than a billion dollars twenty-five years earlier. Most of that growth was driven by five major pharmaceutical companies: Merck, GlaxoSmithKline, Sanofi Aventis, Pfizer, and Novartis. Those are amazing numbers, and they represent a sharp change from the traditional role vaccines played in public health and pharmaceutical manufacturing.

Until late in the twentieth century, the American vaccine business was a low-profit, fragmented industry made up of small, commercial enterprises and divisions of state public health departments. Smallpox, for which the original vaccine was created, had been conquered; polio was driven out of the United States and in retreat elsewhere in the world. The main childhood vaccines besides polio were the combined diphtheria, tetanus, and pertussis shot, which had been around since the 1940s, and the MMR, beginning in the 1970s. In the go-go pharmaceutical world, vaccine production was a sleepy backwater.

On a personal note, both of us grew up in the heart of the baby boom; both of us had measles, mumps, chicken pox, and German measles (rubella). And both of us got just five vaccines—diphtheria, pertussis, tetanus, live-virus polio, and smallpox (now eradicated).

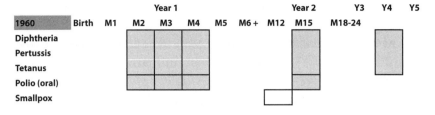

Things didn't change much in the 1970s except for the arrival of individual measles, mumps, and rubella shots.

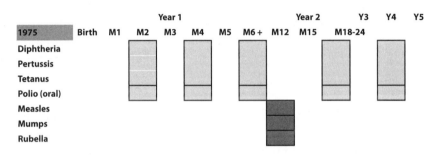

One could argue—we would—that the major childhood illnesses were largely under control.

But in the late 1980s, the business underwent a marked transformation into a high-profit, high-technology growth industry powered by the world's top, multinational pharmaceutical companies. This transformation coincided with the passage by Congress in 1986 of the National Childhood Vaccine Injury Act (NCVIA) and the liability protections it put in place.

In brief, the pediatricians and vaccine manufacturers—who had been threatening to pull out of the business under a barrage of consumer lawsuits—won immunity from liability. You couldn't sue the companies directly anymore, the way you could sue a tire company for making defective tires that led to blowouts and car crashes. Instead, every vaccine recipient pays a 75-cent surcharge that goes into a fund. You now have to take your case to a new vaccine "court"—really an administrative proceeding run by the Department of Health and Human Services, the same department that approves vaccines (the

FDA), recommends their use (the CDC), and vouches for their safety (both).

You have to submit to new and restrictive rules of evidence that prevent "discovery" of potentially incriminating drug company documents (the Wyeth DTP memo would never have surfaced in vaccine "court," for example), agree to keep the proceedings secret, and settle for what in many cases is a small amount of money after many years of litigation. In theory, you could take your case to federal court if you didn't like the outcome—as allowed in other administrative proceedings, like disputes over Social Security Disability benefits. But that avenue of escape was effectively closed recently by a US Supreme Court decision, uniquely cutting off claims of vaccine injury from any real chance to be heard by the regular court system—and a jury.

At the time, the creation of the vaccine "court" seemed like a good idea even to many of those concerned about vaccine safety. One person who expressed doubts, President Ronald Reagan, said, "Although the goal of compensating those persons is a worthy one, the program has . . . serious deficiencies." Among his concerns was the precedent of indemnifying private companies from liability. Nonetheless, Reagan signed the legislation.

The vaccine manufacturers were off and running. First up: Hib vaccine—recommended at 18 months in 1988 and moved up to two months in 1990—and hepatitis B vaccine starting at birth in 1991. Both vaccines contained thimerosal—half ethylmercury by weight—as a preservative. Vaccination rates for the risky, mercury-containing DTP shot also shot up, as pediatricians were emboldened by the new law. Suddenly, infants were getting almost triple the amount of mercury in the first year of life.

For those born in 1988 or later, the risk of autism soared. That was the inflection point for a global rise of autism. In worldwide data sets, "we found that an increase in autism disorder cumulative incidence began about [the birth cohort years] 1988-1989," according to the National Health and Environmental Effects Research Laboratory.

"Although the debate about the nature of increasing autism continues," they added, "the potential for this increase to be real and involve exogenous [external] environmental stressors exists."

In other words, to borrow novelist Joseph Heller's useful title, *Something Happened*. Autism suddenly spiked from a rare and strange affliction into today's 1-in-68 epidemic.

SINCE 1990, AUTISM RATES HAVE EXPLODED: SOMETHING NEW AND TERRIBLE IS HAPPENING TO A GENERATION OF CHILDREN

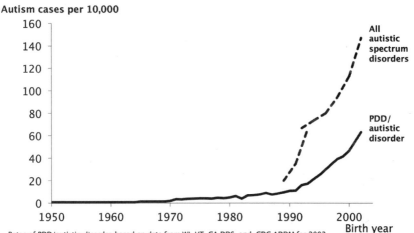

Autism cases per 10,000

Rates of PDD/autistic disorder based on data from WI, UT, CA DDS, and, CDC ADDM for 2002
Rates for all Autism Spectrum Disorder based on surveys of 8-year-olds: MN from 1989–93 and CDC ADDM network from 1992–2002

A 2013 study in Minneapolis found that 1 in every 31 white children—in other words, about one child per typical elementary school classroom—had autism.

Was the intention of NCVIA really to make the world safe for vaccine profits and expose families to greater risk of injury of wildly different types from an explosion in childhood vaccines? Certainly no, but we believe that has been the outcome.

Confirmation comes from data compiled by Gayle DeLong, a professor at Baruch College in Manhattan, who studied vaccines approved by the FDA after "delitigation"—the removal of vaccine-injury claims from civil courts and juries. She describes creation of the vaccine "court" as "a social experiment in the effect of delitigation on product safety" and concludes, "Vaccine safety decreases after consumers are not able to sue vaccine manufacturers."

Not only were vaccines licensed after 1988 linked with twice as many adverse events as those licensed earlier, but the post-1988 vaccines were more likely to cause serious problems than catching the disease itself in the year *before* the vaccine was licensed. Nor were the new vaccines targeted at more serious diseases than existing vaccines, which might justify a higher rate of adverse events.

DeLong based her study in part on the Vaccine Adverse Events Reporting System (VAERS) that began in 1990. Thousands of problems linked to vaccines began popping up. A report from 1992 for a one-year-old boy states: "Patient received MMR vaccination (mumps-measles-rubella) and experienced fever, autistic behaviors, encephalitic condition, began to tune out; sound sensitivity, hand-flapping, wheel-spinning, nighttime sweats, appetite increase."

The child's diagnoses included autism, encephalopathy (brain injury), mental retardation, personality disorder, and speech disorder.

Another early report, in 1994, came from a doctor in California: "There are currently 10 cases of autism in children who received DPT/OPV/MMR at 15-18 months." (OPV means oral polio vaccine, which is no longer used in the United States.)

Reports of a single case or a small cluster are one thing. But not long after the vaccine schedule began expanding, frontline medical professionals started noticing a disturbing change in the children they were seeing day in and day out. A school nurse in Missouri, Patti White, told a House Government Reform subcommittee on June 6, 1999:

> We continually see more and more damaged children entering our schools, and are very concerned that a major portion of that damage may be due to the hepatitis B vaccine's assault on the newborn neurological and immune system.
>
> For the past three or four years our school districts have noted a significant increase in the number of children entering school with developmental disorders, learning disabilities, "attention deficit disorders" and/or serious chronic illness such as diabetes, "asthma," and seizure disorder.

Each of the past four years has been worse than the year before. The census of ill children seen in our health rooms each day has increased by 300 percent in only four years.

A month later, the CDC and the American Academy of Pediatrics urged manufacturers to phase out mercury from childhood vaccines, including hep B, saying there was a "theoretical risk" but no actual evidence of harm. They also temporarily delayed the timing of the shot from birth to six months, which was since reversed.

Another frontline health professional, Dr. Elizabeth Mumper of Lynchburg, Va., began observing a similar phenomenon—a sudden and sizable change for the worse in the overall health of the children in her pediatric practice. Ultimately, Mumper came to suspect the increasing number of childhood vaccinations in the 1990s, and particularly thimerosal—the mercury-based preservative—as a potential cause or trigger.

"In the mid-1990s, I had a general intuitive sense, as a clinician who's walked into rooms with thousands of patients, that children were sicker," she told us. "When I asked myself what I was seeing, I realized I was seeing more development problems, more stuttering, more speech and language issues, more autism, and lots more ADHD [attention deficit hyperactivity disorder]. I was seeing more asthma, more eczema—all those sort of autoimmune allergic conditions.

"I started having more diabetic patients. In this very small practice—I've only got several thousand patients—I had four insulin-dependent diabetics, and they tend to be younger, one diagnosed as young as 16 months old. The incidence of diabetes used to be something like one in 2,000 kids several decades ago.

"As a clinician, I think we shouldn't get hung up on questions like, 'Is this really autism?' or 'Is it Asperger's [a milder variation]?' or have we broadened the definition and included more neurologically damaged kids? The question should be: What has happened to 1 in 6 children in America that both the CDC and the American Academy of Pediatrics acknowledge have a neurodevelopmental disability?"

Mumper has since changed her recommended vaccination schedule and says she is seeing far fewer health problems in her patients; we'll revisit her in Part III.

Schoolteachers have also noticed. While endless debates revolve around classroom size, teacher tenure, "teaching to the test," and other supposed ills of modern American education, those may not be the central problem.

"It's like a mental institution," said a teacher from the Midwest who has taught lower primary grades for twenty-five years. "At any given time you can hear screams coming from down the hallway. It never ends." Asked what's the matter with these kids, he replied: "Different kinds of things—emotional issues, behavior issues, learning issues . . . No girls, all boys. Kids who are just out of control, throwing furniture against the wall, banging their heads, running down the hallway."

"Does it change the way you teach?" we asked. "We don't teach anymore. It stops us from teaching." It didn't used to be this way, he said.

Worldwide data routinely pick up the decline of competitiveness. "Our scores are stagnant. We're not seeing any improvement for our 15-year-olds," Jack Buckley, commissioner at the National Center for Education Statistics, the research arm of the Education Department, told the *Washington Post*. "But our ranking is slipping because a lot of these other countries are improving."

"The U.S. was slotted between the Slovak Republic and Lithuania in the overall results, two spots behind Russia," NPR reported.

By the mid-1990s, the CDC was quietly—very quietly—noticing at least one problem: autism. Marshalyn Yeargin-Allsopp, the CDC's lead autism epidemiologist, said in a speech in 2005: "About ten years ago, we began to hear concerns from around the country that people were seeing more cases of autism." That would be 1995, the same time Patti White and Elizabeth Mumper were making their troubling observations.

VACCINATIONS HAVE SERIOUS RISKS

FROM ITS BEGINNING IN 1988, the VICP has reluctantly compensated indisputable cases of vaccine injury, paying out $2.8 billion even as it resolutely barred the door against autism—one judge famously sneering that, as in Alice in Wonderland, it was "necessary to believe six impossible things before breakfast" to accept an autism-vaccine link.

Several thousand suits alleging such damage were consolidated into one, and ultimately the "special masters" who rule on vaccine cases turned them all down, denouncing the idea that vaccines could possibly trigger a cascade of events that led to autism.

But this wall of denial has begun to crumble. First, it turned out that the government had in fact conceded a link between vaccine damage and autism—in a child named Hannah Poling. The government claimed she had a rare pre-existing mitochondrial disorder that played a role, but the vaccine could just as easily have triggered the problem.

"The funny thing is," said correspondent Alisyn Camerota on Fox News after the Poling case was reported, "no one is saying that vaccines really created autism, so it's . . . they use this very fishy legal language: It didn't cause it, it resulted in it."

Hannah's father, Jon, a Johns Hopkins neurologist, subsequently commented: "I wouldn't have believed it until it happened to me. To be honest with you, as a doctor, until it happened to me, until I saw the regression, until I saw a normal 18 month old toddler descend into autism, I wouldn't have believed it was possible."

...he study, "Unanswered Questions From the Vaccine In-
...mpensation Program: A Review of Compensated Cases of
...e-Induced Brain Injury," showed that in many such cases, the
...dren also have the behavioral diagnosis of autism. The judges in-
...sted that vaccines couldn't, didn't, and wouldn't cause the disorder
even as their own case files show that close to half of vaccine injury
awards went to children with autism.

According to the peer-reviewed 2011 study: "The VICP has compensated approximately 2,500 claims of vaccine injury since the in-
ception of the program. This study found 83 cases of acknowledged
vaccine-induced brain damage that included autism, a disorder that
affects speech, social communication and behavior. In 21 published
cases of the Court of Federal Claims, which administers the VICP,
the Court stated that the petitioners had autism or described autism unambiguously. In 62 remaining cases, the authors identified
settlement agreements where Health and Human Services (HHS)
compensated children with vaccine-induced brain damage, who also
have autism or an autism spectrum disorder. . . .

"The investigation shows that the VICP has been compensating cases of vaccine-induced brain damage associated with autism
for more than twenty years. This investigation suggests that officials at HHS, the Department of Justice and the Court of Federal
Claims may have been aware of this association but failed to pub-
licly disclose it."

Even spokesmen for the program have a hard time dodging the
truth. In an e-mail to the authors of a 2014 law review article, David
Bowman, a spokesman for the Health Resources and Services Administration, said the court "has not compensated any cases based upon
autism alone in the absence of sudden serious brain illness after vaccination." Well, that's the case we're making: Autism does occur after
sudden serious brain illness—encephalopathy—following vaccination.

Rolf Hazlehurst, whose son Yates was one of the test cases for
vaccine injury that the court threw out, has written that "in reality,
the Vaccine Act placed the national vaccine program including vaccine safety under the control of the pharmaceutical industry and
took away the right of the people to legally question vaccine safety
in a court of law."

Consider the case of another child named Hannah—Hannah Bruesewitz, who "hours after a diphtheria-pertussis-tetanus vaccine, developed catastrophic brain injury and a lifelong seizure disorder," according to the Elizabeth Birt Center for Autism Law and Advocacy.

"The only plausible explanation for the harm to Hannah was her vaccine," the center said. "Indeed, many other children were injured by the same vaccine lot, yet the Vaccine Injury Compensation Program, the only court where Hannah could bring her claim, denied compensation after years of litigation. Now the Supreme Court tells Hannah and her family that there is no courtroom in the country in which she can obtain justice and compensation for the years of care ahead that she needs."

If a case as clear as Hannah Bruesewitz's was rejected, no wonder parents of vaccine-injured children can end up feeling alone, abandoned by their doctors and public health officials who had glibly assured them that the risk of vaccine injury was infinitesimal and, if it did occur, would be compensated quickly and generously.

The third problem with the soaring vaccine schedule is that vaccines contain multiple chemicals that are not proven safe to inject in anyone, let alone infants, let alone repeatedly, let alone in combination.

These fall into several categories including preservatives, the most controversial of which is the organic mercury compound, thimerosal. You could write a book on this topic—in fact, we did. Called *The Age of Autism: Mercury, Medicine, and a Man-made Epidemic*, it traces the hidden role of mercury in a whole range of disorders, from the worst form of syphilis to many of Freud's hysteria patients to the first cases of autism.

Those eleven cases, described by a Johns Hopkins psychiatrist in 1943, had striking family connections to the first uses of ethylmercury in medicine, forestry, and plant pathology. We've made, we believe, an irrefutable case that autism began in the 1930s when these ethylmercury compounds were first commercialized, then exploded when more mercury-containing vaccines were added around 1990.

The CDC has a strange and dubious history of investigating concerns about thimerosal. In the late 1990s, Congress ordered the FDA to investigate mercury in medical products. To their horror, agency officials realized they had been "asleep at the switch," as one put it—as the number of vaccines containing mercury rose after 1988, the amount to which an infant would be exposed soared past levels established by safety guidelines.

The CDC, which had recommended those vaccines, set about conducting studies on whether vaccine mercury was causing a rise in autism. Their first data set showed exactly that—children with the highest exposures to mercury in the first month of life were seven to eleven times more likely to develop autism (they did two different analyses) than those with the lowest exposure. CDC officials, according to e-mails and transcripts, were stunned. But rather than sounding the immediate alarm, they set about burying the truth under mounds of bogus epidemiology, betraying the American public whose children they were sworn to protect.

Hear this well: These people should not be entrusted with your infant.

But thimerosal is not the only toxic metal in childhood vaccines. Another is aluminum, used as what's called an adjuvant to boost the immune-stimulating quality of the vaccine. Aluminum has been implicated in a number of serious illnesses, including Alzheimer's disease, and its presence in childhood vaccines remains deeply concerning.

Other compounds in vaccines include formaldehyde, sodium borate, and polysorbate 80, an emulsifier. In the hepatitis B vaccine, remnants of the yeast used to grow the antigen—the molecule that induces immune response—end up in the vaccine, and anyone allergic to yeast is advised not to get the vaccine—although how a newborn baby would know that is a mystery.

Are these compounds safe? Who knows. When safety studies are done, the comparison made is often between the vaccine as used in your pediatrician's office compared with the same vaccine minus only the antigen. In other words, the standard vaccine is tested against the same chemicals—aluminum, formaldehyde, yeast, and mercury, depending on the vaccine—in that vaccine rather than what should be used, a simple saline (salt) solution. This makes it impossible to know if any of those compounds is dangerous in itself, in combination with the vaccine antigen, or when given at the same time as antigens or chemicals in other shots. This is one reason we say safety studies are inadequate.

Beyond the vaccine itself and the chemicals intentionally put into it, there is the matter of what are called "adventitious agents"—such as viruses or viral particles that come from substances, including live-animal tissue, used to grow the vaccines. There is human DNA in some vaccines that comes from aborted fetal tissue used to produce them, as well as animal proteins from eggs, pigs, and other creatures used to create vaccine strains.

Most notorious is SV-40, so named because it was the fortieth simian virus identified in monkey-kidney cells, a cancer-causing substance discovered belatedly in the oral polio vaccine. Although that vaccine is no longer in use in the US, it's possible that tens of millions of baby boomers that received it from the 1960s through the 1990s are infected with what some scientists consider a ticking time bomb.

Also controversial was the discovery of porcine (pig) viruses in the current rotavirus vaccines, viruses that cause wasting disease in pigs. These vaccines in turn had replaced one shown to cause fatal cases of intussusception, in which the bowel folds in on itself. (There have been similar reports from the new vaccines.)

Yet every parent is prodded to get the rotavirus vaccine and its follow-ups for every child, for a disease that is simply not a significant health risk in the developed world.

By the same token, many of the illnesses for which we now vaccinate were in sharp decline before vaccines to prevent them were introduced. That's clearly the case with measles. Improvements in overall health and our understanding of microbes made them much less common even *without* the advent of vaccines. So they perhaps deserve some credit, but not all of it, and not as much as is stoked in the popular imagination.

On the other hand, this argument can go too far. Some vaccine critics argue that polio, for instance, was not eradicated in the United States by the Salk and Sabin vaccines. They say the disease was simply reclassified as "flaccid paralysis" and objective-case reporting was deliberately suppressed.

We don't buy it. The epidemiological evidence is clear that the incidence of polio was wiped out, or at least substantially reduced, by the vaccine.

Utopias, including ones free of disease, are frequently mirages. In the overzealous search for perfect protection, the public health establishment has forgotten the motto of doctors everywhere: First, do no harm.

As John Stone, a contributing editor to our web site, wrote: "The problem is that vaccines are neither as safe or effective as government and health officials say. They aren't properly tested or monitored. The manufacturers have effective immunity from prosecution; there are sanctions against ordinary citizens to accept them. Accurate, truthful information is not made available when obtaining consent, which in some states is coercive anyway. If something does go wrong—and it often does—no one will want to hear your side of the story: you will be met with hostility and having to deal with consequences for the rest of your life and beyond. The system has gone wrong."

We fear that in these children and young adults—millennials born in 1988 and since—a new kind of "Generation X" is emerging—x percent suffering from asthma, x percent from juvenile arthritis, x percent from gut problems, or ADHD, or rheumatoid arthritis, or juvenile diabetes, or autism: mostly illnesses of out-of-whack immune systems almost never seen in children until immunizations suddenly started soaring a generation ago.

This did not need to happen, and it does not need to continue. We can protect our children, our families, our neighbors, and our world from serious diseases *and* prevent the kind of disorders that have soared with the CDC's bloated vaccine schedule.

That begins with you, in the next chapter.

Part II:
What You Should Know

CHAPTER 4

MAKING SENSE OF "THE SCHEDULE"

THE CDC NOW RECOMMENDS THAT EVERY CHILD receive sixteen different types of vaccines in sixty-eight doses before their eighteenth birthday.

Alphabetically, those vaccines are for chicken pox, diphtheria, haemophilus influenza B (Hib), hepatitis A, hepatitis B, human papilloma virus (HPV), influenza, measles, meningococcal disease, mumps, pertussis, pneumococcal disease, polio, rotavirus, rubella, and tetanus.

All sixteen vaccines are given more than once. For instance, the hepatitis B shot is routinely given for the first time before a newborn leaves the maternity ward, followed by two more doses by six months.

Counting it all up, the CDC recommends children receive forty-nine vaccine doses by their fifth birthday. After that comes a round of boosters before elementary school, and for older kids, three human papilloma virus vaccines, a combination tetanus-diphtheria-pertussis shot, and two meningococcal vaccines. Plus an influenza vaccination every year.

That adds up to sixty-eight doses by the time a child turns eighteen, not to mention two shots while the mother is carrying the fetus. By any reckoning, that's a lot—and a lot to keep track of—as you can see from this eye-tiring chart from the CDC.

Figure 1. Recommended immunization schedule for persons aged 0 through 18 years – United States, 2014.

(FOR THOSE WHO FALL BEHIND OR START LATE, SEE THE CATCH-UP SCHEDULE [FIGURE 2]).

These recommendations must be read with the footnotes that follow. For those who fall behind or start late, provide catch-up vaccination at the earliest opportunity as indicated by the green bars in Figure 1. To determine minimum intervals between doses, see the catch-up schedule (Figure 2). School entry and adolescent vaccine age groups are in bold.

Vaccine	Birth	1 mo	2 mos	4 mos	6 mos	9 mos	12 mos	15 mos	18 mos	19-23 mos	2-3 yrs	4-6 yrs	7-10 yrs	11-12 yrs	13-15 yrs	16-18 yrs
Hepatitis B[1] (HepB)	1st dose	←2nd dose→			←——— 3rd dose ———→											
Rotavirus[2] (RV) RV1 (2-dose series); RV5 (3-dose series)			1st dose	2nd dose	See footnote 2											
Diphtheria, tetanus, & acellular pertussis[3] (DTaP: <7 yrs)			1st dose	2nd dose	3rd dose		←———— 4th dose ————→					5th dose				
Tetanus, diphtheria, & acellular pertussis[4] (Tdap: ≥7 yrs)														(Tdap)		
Haemophilus influenzae type b[5] (Hib)			1st dose	2nd dose	See footnote 5		3rd or 4th dose, See footnote 5									
Pneumococcal conjugate[6] (PCV13)			1st dose	2nd dose	3rd dose		←———— 4th dose ————→									
Pneumococcal polysaccharide[6] (PPSV23)																
Inactivated poliovirus[7] (IPV) (<18 yrs)			1st dose	2nd dose	←——————— 3rd dose ———————→							4th dose				
Influenza[8] (IIV; LAIV) 2 doses for some. See footnote 8					Annual vaccination (IIV only)						Annual vaccination (IIV or LAIV)					
Measles, mumps, rubella[9] (MMR)							←—— 1st dose ——→					2nd dose				
Varicella[10] (VAR)							←—— 1st dose ——→					2nd dose				
Hepatitis A[11] (HepA)							←— 2-dose series. See footnote 11 —→									
Human papillomavirus[12] (HPV2: females only; HPV4: males and females)														(3-dose series)		
Meningococcal[13] (Hib-MenCY ≥ 6 weeks; MenACWY-D ≥9 mos; MenACWY-CRM ≥ 2 mos)							See footnote 13							1st dose		Booster

Legend:
- Range of recommended ages for all children
- Range of recommended ages for catch-up immunization
- Range of recommended ages for certain high-risk groups
- Range of recommended ages during which catch-up is encouraged and for certain high-risk groups
- Not routinely recommended

This schedule includes recommendations in effect as of January 1, 2014. Any dose not administered at the recommended age should be administered at a subsequent visit, when indicated and feasible. The use of a combination vaccine generally is preferred over separate injections of its equivalent component vaccines. Vaccination providers should consult the relevant Advisory Committee on Immunization Practices (ACIP) statement for detailed recommendations, available online at http://www.cdc.gov/vaccines/hcp/acip-recs/index.html. Clinically significant adverse events that follow vaccination should be reported to the Vaccine Adverse Event Reporting System (VAERS) online (http://www.vaers.hhs.gov) or by telephone (800-822-7967). Suspected cases of vaccine preventable diseases should be reported to the state or local health department. Additional information, including precautions and contraindications for vaccination, is available from CDC online (http://www.cdc.gov/vaccines/recs/vac-admin/contraindications.htm) or by telephone (800-CDC-INFO [800-232-4636]).

This schedule is approved by the Advisory Committee on Immunization Practices (http://www.cdc.gov/vaccines/acip), the American Academy of Pediatrics (http://www.aap.org), the American Academy of Family Physicians (http://www.aafp.org), and the American College of Obstetricians and Gynecologists (http://www.acog.org).

To start making sense of this, we've created our own, simplified version of the vaccine schedule for just the preschool years, listing each vaccine and booster at its *earliest* recommended age (vaccines added since the baby-boom era are in a darker shade). This is the way many pediatricians give the injections—as soon, and as many, as possible. At six months, for instance, a child could receive nine vaccinations—hep B, rotavirus, DTaP (three vaccines in one shot), haemophilus influenza B (Hib), pneumococcal, polio, and flu.

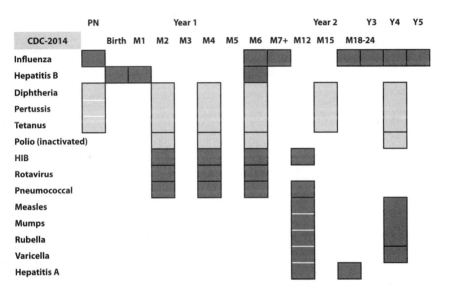

So that's the schedule. But what, exactly, is the rationale for each vaccine? Everyone knows about polio, which can paralyze and kill you, and chicken pox, which gives you a few spots, but can anyone describe the diseases and dangers between those two extremes? How about just the four H's—hep A, hep B, Hib, and HPV?

Anyone?

And how well does each vaccine prevent the disease it targets? On the downside of the equation, how risky is each vaccine, both separately and when given with other vaccines? Do the rewards outweigh the risks—for your child?

THE SIX TYPES OF VACCINES: REWARDS AND RISKS

AS WE'VE OUTLINED IN PART I, THESE ARE QUESTIONS YOU HAVE A RIGHT—in fact, a responsibility—to ask and get answered. To help, we've broken down the CDC schedule and put it back together in a more thematic way, based on the type of disease each vaccine is intended to prevent. The vaccines then fall naturally into six clusters:

1. **Cancer vaccines:** hepatitis B and HPV, designed to prevent chronic infections that may lead to cancer.

2. **Live-virus vaccines:** measles, mumps, rubella, and chicken pox, all weakened live-virus vaccines.

3. **Influenza vaccine:** both the seasonal flu shot (usually three strains at once) and shots for specific strains like H1N1.

4. **Enteric vaccines:** rotavirus, polio, and hepatitis A to prevent viral infections that enter the body through the gastrointestinal tract.

5. **Early bacterial vaccines:** diphtheria, pertussis, tetanus; these are the oldest vaccines still given and they were put together in the 1940s in the first combination vaccines.

6. **Bacterial meningitis vaccines:** Hib, pneumococcal, and meningococcal, all bacteria that can cause meningitis (and

in the case of *streptococcus pneumoniae*, illnesses like pneumonia and other invasive infections).

For each vaccine, we'll ask eight questions—four about the potential rewards of getting the vaccine, and four about the possible risks, scoring each vaccine on each question from -5 to +5. The total score, positive or negative, is the vaccine's Reward-Risk Rating. The higher the score, the better the balance of reward over risk, with all of our judgments based on extensive research and analysis as well as many years of experience in the vaccine safety controversies. In several cases, we have cited data collected by Gayle DeLong, a leading vaccine safety advocate and professor at Baruch College in Manhattan.

You'll notice that our Reward-Risk Rating places only four vaccines above the break-even line for reward over risk. Two are at zero, and ten are in minus territory. Where you as a consumer will draw your own lines, and how you will weigh the rewards and benefits of each vaccine, may be different from ours. We have based this judgment on an honest and objective evaluation of the real likelihood of catching or spreading the diseases, the severity of the illness, and, of course, risks from the vaccines themselves.

We want to emphasize one important thing. Our Reward-Risk Rating is only an index, not a recommendation; we don't assign our eight categories any kind of differential weighting but instead leave that balancing act up to you.

The 3 R Chart
Reward-Risk Rating

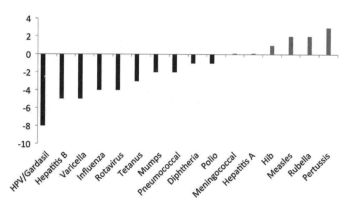

Do remember, vaccines are described by no less than the Supreme Court of the United States as "unavoidably unsafe." Any vaccine—like any medical intervention—can cause an adverse event no matter how careful a patient, parent, or pediatrician is trying to be. You should bear in mind the unpredictable risk of an "idiosyncratic" reaction as you weigh your decisions and be prepared to get treatment and documentation.

In Part III, we'll help you implement the schedule you choose, take additional steps to avoid vaccine injury, and identify and report a problem if it does occur.

Risk Reward Rating summary

BENEFITS	Cancer		Flu	Enteric		Live viral					Bacterial				Meningitis	
	Hep B	HPV		Rotavirus	Polio	Measles	Mumps	Rubella	Varicella	Hepatitis A	Diphtheria	Pertussis	Tetanus	Hib	Pneumococcal	Meningococcal
1. How bad is the disease?	5	1	1	0	4	3	1	2	1	1	4	4	5	5	4	3
2. How much am I protecting others?	0	3	2	3	0	4	4	5	-5	1	1	5	0	1	1	1
3. What is the risk of infection?	1	4	3	4	0	0	1	0	1	1	1	2	1	1	1	0
4. How effective is the vaccine?	1	1	1	2	3	4	1	4	4	4	3	2	3	3	1	2
RISKS																
1. How bad are the side effects?	-2	-5	-4	-5	-2	-1	-1	-1	-1	-1	-3	-3	-3	-1	-1	-1
2. What is the risk of chronic disease and death?	-5	-5	-4	-4	-3	-4	-4	-4	-2	-3	-4	-4	-4	-3	-3	-2
3. What the risk of this vaccine in combination with others?	-1	-2	-2	-2	-2	-4	-4	-4	-3	-2	-3	-3	-3	-3	-3	-1
4. Are there other ways of preventing/treating the disease?	-4	-5	-1	-2	-1	0	0	0	0	-1	0	0	-2	-2	-2	-2
Total score	-5	-8	-4	-2	-1	2	-2	2	-5	0	-1	3	-3	1	-2	0

CHAPTER 6

THE CANCER VACCINES

- Hepatitis B (hep B)
- Human papillomavirus (HPV)

CANCER KILLS MORE THAN HALF A MILLION AMERICANS EVERY YEAR, and the effort to conquer it has been disheartening—a record of "meager progress," as *Newsweek* magazine put it, since Richard Nixon declared the nation's "War on Cancer" in 1971.

For many decades, the National Cancer Institute—established in 1937 by President Roosevelt—has been the agency at the forefront of the so-called War on Cancer. Perhaps the earliest inspiration for both the cancer war and the development of cancer-preventing vaccines began during the 1960s, when NCI researchers first started looking in earnest at viruses as a potential cause of cancer. In 1961, NCI leaders created the Laboratory of Viral Oncology to begin the search for cancer-causing viruses; in 1962 the Human Cancer Virus Task Force was first convened; and by the end of the decade, enthusiasm over this research was part of the scientific momentum that persuaded President Nixon to launch the War on Cancer in 1971.

Unfortunately for Nixon's legacy, and for most subsequent cancer victims, the War on Cancer has famously failed to find a cure for cancer or to validate theories of viral causation in the vast majority of human cancers.

More people actually die of cancer now than they did when the War on Cancer was declared, and while there are explanations—the increase and aging of the population and more environmental toxins, etc.—it is not an encouraging trend.

On the face of it, vaccines that promise to *prevent* certain types of cancer look like a bright spot in this rather dismal portrait. The devil, as usual, is in the details. A vaccine that prevented cancer with no serious side effects would be a total winner—a 20 out of 20 on our Reward-Risk Rating. But the current picture of cancer vaccines is a good deal more clouded.

As of 2014, the CDC recommends two such vaccines. One, on the childhood immunization schedule since 1991, targets the hepatitis B virus that can lead to liver cancer. The second vaccine, among the CDC's most recent recommendations, made in 2006, is designed to protect against the human papillomavirus that may lead to cervical and possibly other cancers.

Hepatitis B Vaccine

While the intent to prevent cancer is commendable, many parents and activists see the hep B vaccine as the poster child for a bloated enterprise that has gone too far—jamming as many shots into babies as soon as possible to prevent every conceivable disease risk, rather than warding off real and present dangers.

In a discussion thread on a *New York Times* column in 2014, a commenter named Mary wrote:

> The risk of all diseases is not the same and until the recommended American vaccine schedule is reconsidered, parents will continue to resist. It is one thing to protect your child and neighbors against measles, pertussis, and other often dangerous diseases. But in addition, parents are now expected to immunize children against Hepatitis B on their first day of life. Who does this benefit? Which children are at risk of Hep B or at risk of spreading it? Are there reliable studies showing that the vaccine is 100% or 99% [effective] for a newborn?

A mother named Cynthia Parker commented: "My baby was given the hep B shot at the hospital at birth without permission, and even though I'd told her pedi [pediatrician] I absolutely did not want her to get that vaccine: I was negative for hep B, and I had read the vaccine often caused autism. So they gave it to her anyway, and she reacted the way many thousands of children have . . . with four days and nights of endless, inconsolable screaming, vaccine encephalitis."

Those two comments make the case against hepatitis B vaccine for babies: Although the illness can be serious, is the vaccine really necessary for the overwhelming majority of children, especially when those at risk—infants born to the small percentage of mothers infected with hepatitis B—can easily be identified and protected? Despite official claims that the shot is as safe as mother's milk, some children clearly react badly, and some have died following vaccination. Nor is there convincing evidence that the immunity conferred lasts long enough to matter—when a child reaches adolescence and beyond.

Hepatitis B is a viral infection of the liver transmitted by bodily fluids, especially blood. It usually clears up in a few weeks, and many people don't notice any symptoms at all. But in a small percentage of cases, the initial infection can fail to clear and the liver can become chronically infected. That can lead to liver disease, liver cancer, and death.

Newborns of infected mothers can be exposed during birth, and are likelier to develop the chronic form. Fortunately, a routine test during pregnancy will detect hepatitis B in the mother, and immediate treatment with immunoglobulin can prevent the disease in the child, while vaccination of the newborn may add an extra preventive benefit, cutting off the disease transmission process before it starts, or so the theory goes.

In the United States, fewer than 1 percent of mothers are infected with hep B. Otherwise, the risk for infants and children is negligible. Sexual contact and intravenous drug use are the primary ways to contract hepatitis B; healthcare workers are at risk from exposure by infected patients, especially through accidental needle sticks. Those risks, obviously, are years away from the maternity ward, and there is plenty of time to ward them off.

So why vaccinate every single newborn in the United States? Public health officials make vague claims about the risk of "horizontal" transmission from child to child in day care settings or in households where someone is infected. But when push comes to shove, officials acknowledge it's because newborn babies are a classic captive audience—the phrase "get 'em while they're young" is certainly apt.

When the CDC's Advisory Committee on Immunization Practices recommended the shot for all newborns in 1991, the committee said: "In the United States, most infections occur among adults and adolescents. Efforts to vaccinate persons in the major risk groups have had limited success. For example, programs directed at injecting drug users failed to motivate them to receive three doses of vaccine. . . . In the United States it has become evident that HBV transmission cannot be prevented through vaccinating only the groups at high risk of infection. . . . In the long term, universal infant vaccination would eliminate the need for vaccinating adolescents and high-risk adults."

But what about the risk to infants right now from a vaccine aimed at protecting against their possible future behavior? Despite official dismissals, they appear to be very real.

A tragic case in point: Lyla Rose Belkin, the daughter of prominent Wall Street analyst Michael Belkin, died in 1998 at the age of five weeks, about fifteen hours after receiving her second booster. "She was never ill before receiving the hepatitis B shot that afternoon," Belkin testified before Congress in 1999. "At her final feeding that night, she was extremely agitated, noisy, and feisty—and then she fell asleep suddenly and stopped breathing. The autopsy ruled out choking, the NY Medical Examiner ruled her death Sudden Infant Death Syndrome (SIDS)."

Typically, the mainstream medical community treats this as coincidence. In another case, Ian Gromowski of Wisconsin got his hep B shot at less than a week old, even though he had a slight fever. For Ian, sadly, the injury from the vaccine was glaringly obvious. "Within twelve hours of his vaccination he had the rash, within twenty-four hours the severe thrombocytopenia set in, and then he was in a fatal state from then on," his mother, Deanna, wrote. He died forty-seven days after the shot. Despite the unmistakably sequential relationship between the administration of the vaccine and the highly unusual reactions, the official response was again denial: "No doctors, nurses, staff would even consider the vaccination as the source."

Several studies also point to long-term dangers from the vaccine. Researchers at the State University of New York at Stony Brook found that the risk for autism triples in newborn baby boys given the hep B vaccination. An earlier study by the same researchers found the chances of being in special education classes were nine times greater for boys vaccinated with hep B than boys who were not.

In 2009, a research team reported that exposure to a birth dose of a hepatitis B vaccine caused significant delays in the development of several survival reflexes in male rhesus macaque monkeys. Those macaques took more than twice as long as unexposed monkeys to acquire three standardized skills typically used to measure infant-brain development.

The irony in all this is that the hep B vaccine was heralded as a breakthrough technology in vaccine development: the model of the next-generation, safer and more effective vaccine. And compared to some vaccines that spent their early days incubating in chicken eggs or aborted fetal tissue, hepatitis B vaccination is in fact a relatively advanced product.

Surrounding the hepatitis B virus is a protective envelope that contains proteins called surface antigens. To make the recombinant vaccine, the genetic code for one of those proteins is inserted into a yeast cell, which grows a copy of the molecule. The vaccine triggers the immune system to "remember" the antigen by making disease-fighting cells called antibodies. If the actual virus ever comes knocking, the body will send its defenders to the door.

This new type of vaccine—genetically engineered using recombinant yeast to produce the hepatitis B surface antigen in large volumes—is reflected in the names of the two brands commonly used in the US: Recombivax HB®, manufactured by Merck, and Engerix-B®, from GlaxoSmithKline. The ingredients are similar: Recombivax contains the hep B surface protein, aluminum, yeast proteins, saline, and formaldehyde. Engerix contains those ingredients plus phosphate buffers to stabilize the solution.

One other unique feature of the hep B vaccine: It's the only routine vaccination given at birth (the influenza vaccine and Tdap are recommended during pregnancy, thus exposing the fetus). This can create a special challenge as it is sometimes given in the maternity ward without parental consent. If you choose not to have your child vaccinated at that time, you need to make your wishes clear.

And you need to be vigilant: even if you think your instructions are ironclad, there are many stories like Cynthia Parker's of parents giving verbal orders not to administer the shot, only to realize later that their nurse did it anyway. Our advice: Put it in writing, and make sure someone accompanies the child to any medical procedure. It is worth the extra vigilance.

Reward Factors

Question 1: How bad is the disease?

Bad for baby. This is a serious disease for a baby to get, and if a mother gives it to her newborn infant, that's a heavy burden to bear. As many as nine in ten infants infected with hep B will go on to develop the chronic infection, according to the CDC; the rate drops to 25 to 50 percent among one- to five-year-olds, and plummets to 6 to 10 percent over age five. In chronic infections, 15 to 25 percent of carriers will go on to develop serious liver problems including cirrhosis and liver cancer. For an infected infant, that is a serious risk from a serious disease.

Score: +5

Question 2: Does getting the vaccine help protect others from getting the same illness?

Health officials make large claims for the vaccine, describing the millions of children infected every year in the world. But the truth is that in the United States, today, the risk is small. No, an infant is highly unlikely to have an undetected hep B infection and even less likely to ever spread the disease.

Score: 0

Question 3: What is the risk of infection?

Very low for baby. Unless the mother is infected—which can be determined before birth—the real risk comes from sexual activity and IV drug use years later. Parents who are concerned could still give their child the vaccine by puberty, like the HPV vaccine (see next section).

Public health officials routinely overstate the risks of an infectious disease to create a case for adding a new vaccine and encouraging its adoption. When the hep B vaccine was introduced, the US incidence rate was placed as high as 350,000 even though the actual number of confirmed cases was a fraction of that. Recognizing that these were mostly cases among populations of IV drug users, homosexual men, and prostitutes, health officials also built an alarmist case for a large number of "horizontal transmission" cases in childhood. Out of those 350,000 cases, over 15,000 were claimed to arise in infants.

Truth be told, in the statistical model that was used to generate that inflated estimate, the number of hepatitis cases actually measured in children was less than ten, most of these in ten-year-old girls.

Not surprisingly, now that the vaccine has been securely established on the routine schedule, these estimates have been quietly, but drastically, reduced. CDC now estimates new annual infections at less than 19,000 cases (not much higher than their previous inflated estimate of 16,000 cases in children alone), a number that declined sharply in the 1980s for reasons unrelated to the infant vaccine.

Score: +1

Question 4: How well does the vaccine work?

The CDC says it protects more than 90 percent of those who receive the vaccine from getting the disease. One question is, for how long? Studies have found a lack of antibodies in the blood—signaling an inability to identify and fight off the disease—seven to ten years after vaccination in infancy. The widely respected Cochrane Collaboration reviewed twelve studies on the effectiveness of the vaccine, and found that all "had high risk of bias and the reporting was inconsistent," concluding: "In people not previously exposed to hepatitis B, vaccination has unclear effect on the risk of developing infection, as compared to no vaccination."

In other words, it may not work when it's needed. For a parent evaluating the true preventive benefits of this high-tech vaccine, the compelling evidence for its value is frustatingly hard to find.

Score: +1

Risk Factors

Question 1: What are the vaccine's side effects?

None, according to the CDC. "The hepatitis vaccine is safe," the CDC declares. "Since the vaccine became available in 1982, more than 100 million people have received hepatitis B vaccination in the United States and no serious side effects have been reported." This is clearly propaganda, not science. According to data compiled by vaccine safety advocate Gayle DeLong, a total of 37,108 adverse events after hepatitis B vaccination were reported from 1991 to 2010 to the Vaccine Adverse Event Reporting System, run by the CDC and the Food and Drug Administration. That gives the vaccine an adverse-events-per-immunization-series ratio of 12.31 per 100,000 recipients. A total of 294 deaths were reported, for a ratio of 0.1299. That is *not* nothing, especially given the fact that public health officials acknowledge adverse events are underreported by a factor of ten to one hundred.

According to the vaccine package insert, provided by the manufacturer, the most common reactions—affecting more than 1 percent of patients—are injection-site soreness and swelling, fatigue, weakness, headache, fever, nausea, and diarrhea. Less common reactions include vomiting, dizziness, and low blood pressure. After the vaccine was approved, reactions included a worrisome cluster of neurological events: Guillain-Barré syndrome, multiple sclerosis, seizure, febrile seizure, peripheral neuropathy including Bell's Palsy, herpes zoster, migraine, muscle weakness, and encephalitis. Other studies have detected a risk for juvenile diabetes, which along with other chronic childhood disorders has soared since the new wave of vaccines started pouring over the no-liability dam in 1988.

A big problem is that side effects were not studied adequately before the vaccine was approved: reports on the clinical trials provide little information on the 2,000 to 3,000 newborns who received th. vaccine. In some cases safety reports were based on only four days of follow-up; another study of the VAERS system found 18 deaths but dismissed these as unrelated to the vaccine, even though the people who reported them must have believed there was a possible link.

That's the kind of "evidence" the CDC is using when it says no serious side effects have been reported.

Score: -2

Question 2: What are the risks of chronic/severe illness and death?

A number of parents believe the hep B vaccination killed their children (see above). The Stony Brook studies cited above found heightened risks for autism and the need for special education services in vaccinated boys; this study was largely completed before a phase-out of ethylmercury in the vaccine began in 1999. And the Hewitson primate study, also noted above, showed the birth dose caused significant delays in developing brain and survival instincts of monkeys.

Score: -5

Question 3: What are the consequences of using the vaccine in combination with other vaccines?

The vaccine is given alone to newborns, then again at one to two months, and six to eighteen months. Vaccination at two months, six months, and beyond puts the hep B in a pileup of scheduled shots that means it could interact with other vaccines, a phenomenon that the CDC and drugmakers have failed to study. In particular, the aluminum in the shot is multiplied when given with one or more vaccines that also contain the toxic metal. Mercury-containing flu shots can create interactions with hep B that are far more dangerous than either metal on its own.

Combination hep B shots have been licensed in the United States. These include: Twinrix®, which combines hep B with hep A vaccines;

, which combines DTaP, hep B, and polio vaccines; and a combination of hep B and Hib vaccine.

Question 4: Are there ways to protect against the disease without getting the vaccine?

The main risk for the disease at birth is if the mother is a carrier of the hepatitis B virus and transmits it to the child during the birthing process. If the mother doesn't have hep B, there's no risk, and checking for hep B status while pregnant will help ensure that her infant is safe from hep B as well. If the mother is hep B positive, then the vaccine and/or hep B immunoglobulin after birth would be indicated.

Score: -4

Overall Reward-Risk Rating: -5

The Big Picture: A Vaccine's Rapid Rise

The hep B vaccine is the classic illustration of how liability protection for manufacturers quickly generated huge paydays for new vaccines. In the early 1980s, the hep B vaccine was made from the plasma of people infected with the virus, and the target was generally sexually active gay men and drug abusers—the same group vulnerable to another illness borne by blood and bodily fluids, AIDS. It was a small niche in a sleepy business.

Due to limited supply and fears of contamination, researchers went to work to create a better version. Scottish scientist Kenneth Murray devised the technique of recombining DNA to create a vaccine that allowed large-scale production in the laboratory. The effort was altruistic: Murray, who was knighted for his work, donated his share of the patent proceeds to create a foundation. "I could have taken the money but I don't need to. I don't particularly want a Rolls-Royce," said Murray. CDC epidemiologist Don Francis, one of the heroes of the AIDS epidemic, was a leader in testing the vaccine and recommending it for universal use.

Others did profit—immensely. The new vaccines weres among the first big beneficiaries of the 1986 law that lifted liability from vaccine manufacturers.

GlaxoSmithKline's Engerix B® was approved in Belgium in October of that year, with sales reaching roughly $35 million there just two years later. For SmithKline Biologicals (the ancestor of GSK Biologics, the multibillion-dollar vaccine division of pharmaceutical giant GlaxoSmithKline) it was the company's only vaccine besides the polio vaccine. Introduced in the United States in 1989, sales quickly exceeded $90 million, jumping to $160 million the next year, and to more than $500 million by 1992.

Although Merck didn't regularly break out separate figures for Recombivax®, its high-tech vaccine has followed a similar trajectory. The year before the vaccine act, its total vaccine sales were around $100 million; half a dozen years later, in 1992, they were $500 million or so, and "sales gains [in the Merck Vaccine division] . . . were again led by Recombivax HB," Merck said.

Both companies are now vaccine powerhouses. Merck had sales of $5.5 billion in 2013, while Glaxo reached $5.4 billion—a dramatic rise following the government's decision to recommend every newborn get a shot almost none of them needed. It was a pattern destined to repeat itself.

After NCVIA liability shield went into effect in 1988, new hepatitis B vaccine revenues exploded

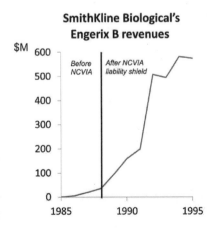

SmithKline Biological's Engerix B revenues

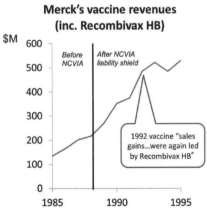

Merck's vaccine revenues (inc. Recombivax HB)

HPV Vaccine

Human papillomavirus (HPV) is actually a family of more than one hundred sexually transmitted virus types, about fifteen of which can cause cervical cancer in women or genital warts in both sexes. Most people who have sex (which is, in fact, most people) eventually become infected—by age fifty, more than four out of five women who have been sexually active are infected.

The infection is usually benign, but according to the CDC, HPV is responsible for virtually all the 12,000 cases of cervical cancer in the United States each year, including 4,000 deaths. Before the advent of the vaccine, recommended in 2006 for girls (and in 2009 for boys), the main line of defense against cervical cancer was the pap smear, which can detect pre-cancerous lesions on the lining of the cervix.

The leading HPV vaccine, Gardasil, contains "virus like particles" that resemble four strains of HPV, types 6, 11, 16, and 18; the first two prevent warts and the last two cervical cancer. (The other vaccine licensed in the US, Cerverix, contains only types 16 and 18, so it can't prevent genital warts and isn't recommended for boys.) These "virus like particles" are synthesized artificially utilizing patented technologies that allow them to closely resemble the authentic proteins in the real virus. Manufacturers and public health officials hope the the vaccine will ward off the large majority of cervical cancer cases.

The key word is "hope." Because cervical cancer is slow to develop—an average time of fifteen years—there is not yet enough evidence to say that the vaccine will actually work. Researchers are at work on updates to the original formula that will include more HPV types. Meanwhile, pap smears remain an effective and necessary final line of defense.

But while its efficacy is yet to be determined, the vaccine's safety profile has been setting off alarm bells. The shot is recommended as a three-dose series at age eleven or twelve, and thousands of teen girls all over the world appear to have been injured by the vaccine—from acute pain and fainting after vaccination to long-term effects including seizures, heart problems, arthritis, and death.

For this reason, the HPV vaccine has gotten some seriously bad press—at least in other countries. In Japan in early 2014, the government withdrew its recommendation of the vaccine for at least a year. This came after a government task force examined 2,000 reports of HPV vaccine injuries in Japan and found 357 of them to be serious.

Nor did the vaccine fare well in comments by a French expert, Dr. Bernard Dalbergue. He stated in April 2014:

> I predict that Gardasil will become the greatest medical scandal of all times because at some point in time, the evidence will add up to prove that this vaccine . . . has absolutely no effect on cervical cancer and that all the very many adverse effects which destroy lives and even kill, serve no other purpose than to generate profit for the manufacturers.

In June 2014, families of girls who alleged they were injured by HPV vaccines met with England's Shadow Minister for Public Health, Luciana Berger MP, and other politicians to describe their experiences.

This news, like so much else contrary to the official line—that all vaccines are safe and effective and essential—failed to penetrate the mainstream media in the United States. Instead, when adverse effects of the HPV vaccine get a high-profile airing in the US, the counterattack is brutal.

On Katie Couric's talk show in December 2013, a segment devoted to the vaccine featured parents and girls who described the harm it triggered—in active teens who got the shot and quickly developed serious illness and even died. Emily Tarsell described her daughter Kristina, who "was previously healthy, had no existing conditions." After the shot, "she did begin to develop some things—'Oh, I have a rash . . . wonder what that's all about. I feel dizzy.' And she reported this within a few days of her third shot and within eighteen days of the Gardasil shot, she was found dead in her bed."

Rosemary Mathis talked about her daughter, Lauren.
Katie: What an ordeal you both have been through. Rosemary, I know that you were frustrated because you felt you were being ignored by the doctors when you had concerns about how Lauren was doing. And then you finally get to a

doctor at Duke. What did that doctor tell you?

Rosemary: The doctor looked through her records, which were probably a foot tall . . . all these medical records and he analyzed everything, ran tests, and he told me that she had a vaccine injury.

Katie: Now, when he said a vaccine injury, he wasn't specific about Gardasil but that's the conclusion you drew?

Rosemary: No he was not, but Gardasil was the only vaccine she had at that time.

Katie: Lauren, tell me what a typical day was like for you when you were going through this because I know, I understand, you were in a great deal of pain.

Lauren: A typical day was mostly spent in bed. If I was able to get up and walk around, I was doing pretty good. Due to the nausea and headaches, the pain really came from . . . a lot was my gall bladder had stopped functioning . . . so that caused a great deal of pain.

The reaction was furious, both on the show's blog, where the reliable assemblage of vaccine-injury deniers (some of them doubtless paid "trolls") weighed in, and in the mainstream media, much of it buoyed by pharmaceutical ads. "There is no 'HPV Vaccine Controversy,'" wrote *Time* magazine. "At least, not when it comes to the injection's safety. And yet, that was the title of the lead segment on Katie Couric's daytime talk show, 'Katie,' this afternoon. The nearly half-hour story, which the program called their 'Big Conversation,' centered around two mothers who believe the vaccine for human papillomavirus (HPV) harmed their daughters."

The pressure grew so intense that Couric finally backtracked. "Following the show, and in fact before it even aired, there was criticism that the program was too anti-vaccine and anti-science, and in retrospect, some of that criticism was valid," Couric wrote on the

Huffington Post. "We simply spent too much tim[e] adverse events that have been reported in very rare the vaccine. More emphasis should have been given t[o] efficacy of the HPV vaccines."

How do you give more emphasis to the safety a[nd] something that is quite evidently unsafe and whose e yet established? And how does compelling evidence o. vaccine injury lead one country to suspend its recommendation and another's political leaders to meet with concerned families, while in the United States even discussing the issue sends a top TV personality (and her network, owned by Disney) running for cover? The answer lies in the hammerlock that pharmaceutical advertising (not allowed in most other developed countries) has over the national media, especially television, with its endless shilling of pills to sleep, focus, cheer up, calm down, have sex, avoid heart attacks while having sex, and overcome the effects of other advertised products. The launch of Gardasil coincided with a "One Less" campaign from Merck that saturated the airwaves and brought the network millions in ad revenue.

Pharma's influence on political decisionmakers also plays a role. Gardasil briefly became an issue in the 2012 presidential campaign when Governor Rick Perry, R-Texas, took heat for trying to mandate the vaccine in his home state after getting a donation from Merck; a former top aide was a lobbyist for the company. The mandate failed, in part because of criticism from conservatives that it might encourage sexual activity by teens.

Another factor is the evolution of the vaccine: Like the hep B vaccine, it grew out of the War on Cancer and, for better or worse, was backed by the full faith and credit of the US government.

In the chapter "License to Kill?" published in the book *Vaccine Epidemic*, we showed how the US government developed the vaccine, profits from its sales, and protects its reputation in the face of growing evidence of harm. Meanwhile, key officials involved in the decisions rotate through a revolving door into private industry.

Now, in California, the state government has taken the decision out of parents' hands: A new law allows children as young as twelve to receive the vaccine without their parents' consent. If adverse events occur, the parents might never relate them to the shots.

case against this vaccine is one of the strongest we have ____; it's the lowest on our Reward-Risk Rating at negative 8. According to a leading scientific critic of HPV vaccines, Dr. Sin Hang Lee, "HPV vaccination is unnecessary and potentially dangerous to some recipients. This is the first vaccine invented by the government, patented by the government, approved by the government, regulated by the government and promoted by the government to prevent an already preventable disease (cervical cancer) 30 years down the road based on using a poorly demarcated, self-reversible surrogate end-point (CIN2/CIN3 lesions) for evaluation of vaccine efficacy, a big scientific fraud. There are no cervical cancer epidemics in any developed countries."

Reward Factors

Question 1: How bad is the disease?

HPV can cause cervical cancer, which can be fatal, as well as genital warts in males and females. (Gardasil®, but not Cervarix®, is also licensed to protect against genital warts and against cancers of the vulva, penis, and anus.) In the vast majority of cases, however, our immune systems fight off the virus.

Score: +1

Question 2: Does getting the vaccine help protect others from getting the same illness?

Yes, vaccination before a person becomes sexually active prevents the spread of the HPV types in the vaccine to another person. This is the argument advanced most strongly by vaccine marketers and the main reason to target boys. But there are cancer-causing strains not included in current vaccines and much that is not known about the dozens of less common HPV strains, including the likelihood that new strains will emerge to take the place of the two to four variants targeted in the vaccines.

Score: +3

Question 3: What is the risk of infection?

High. Most people who are sexually active will be exposed to HPV eventually. According to the CDC, "You can get HPV by having vaginal, anal, or oral sex with someone who has the virus. It is most commonly spread during vaginal or anal sex. HPV can be passed even when an infected person has no signs or symptoms. Anyone who is sexually active can get HPV, even if you have had sex with only one person. You also can develop symptoms years after you have sex with someone who is infected making it hard to know when you first became infected."

Score: +4

Question 4: How well does the vaccine work?

The jury is out and won't return with a verdict for several more years. Because the vaccine was approved in 2006 for girls, and cervical cancer can take decades to develop, conclusive evidence is not available. The theory of efficacy so far is that the vaccine reduces the incidence of precancerous lesions in clinical trials. There is debate over whether reducing these surrogate measures for the actual cancer is truly preventive or whether the actual rate of cancers will remain unchanged.

Score: +1

Risk Factors

Question 1: What are the vaccine's side effects?

They appear to be serious and frequent. According to data compiled by Gayle DeLong, 125.23 adverse events per 100,000 doses of the vaccine have been reported to VAERS, the voluntary government monitoring system. That's the highest ratio of any of the sixteen licen childhood vaccine in the United States. According to another of VAERS, HPV vaccines alone accounted for between cent of all emergency room visits, hospitalizations, extc stays, disabling events, and life-threatening events triggered by vaccines on the childhood-immunization schedule.

Score: -5

Question 2: What are the risks of chronic/severe illness and death?

They appear to be far higher than the government or Merck acknowledge, starting with signs of problems during badly flawed pre-licensure clinical trials.

Score: -5

Question 3: What are the consequences of using the vaccine in combination with other vaccines?

The vaccine is given to older children and might coincide with other vaccines given then like the annual influenza vaccine and the Tdap shot. In some cases, the vaccine is given together with the meningococcal meningitis vaccine, and VAERS reports have indicated especially bad interactions with that vaccine, Menactra®, including convulsions, seizures, spontaneous abortions, and Guillain-Barré Syndrome. Parents can and should ask for it to be given on a separate visit from any other shots the child might be due to receive.

Score: -2

Question 4: Are there ways to protect against the disease without getting the vaccine?

Yes, the CDC notes that using condoms "can lower your chances of getting HPV. But HPV can infect areas that are not covered by a condom—so condoms may not give full protection against getting HPV." The CDC also notes that mutual monogamy with an uninfected partner can prevent infection. In reality, most sexually active adults will be exposed to the virus at some point.

But that does not leave people defenseless. Pap smears are very good at detecting pre-cancerous changes in the lining of the cervix. The cells can be removed. Regular pap smears by themselves are far and away the most effective form of cervical-cancer prevention, widely adopted and easily performed. Despite the widespread marketing campaigns surrounding Gardasil, public health officials still strongly recommend continuing pap smears and cervical examinations.

Score: -5

Reward-Risk Ratio: -8.

The Big Picture: The No-Placebo Effect

News that the HPV vaccine appears to be far more dangerous in practice than in clinical trials shouldn't surprise anyone familiar with the way those trials were performed. It's a problem that goes to the heart of how vaccines are tested before being administered.

There are two core measurements in any clinical trial: efficacy and safety. For efficacy—how well it works—it's important to measure the response of the active ingredient, and one could make an argument to isolate that ingredient in the trial design to make sure it confers a sufficient degree of immune response. In safety, however, it's important to measure the entire vaccine formulation. After all, the intended recipient wouldn't be exposed to injection of any of the vaccine ingredients without getting the shots.

The gold standard in safety assessments is to compare the vaccine to a placebo—a biologically inert substance, often a saline solution (saltwater). That provides a clear measure of whether some element of the vaccine—either on its own or with other components of the shot—is triggering a problem that wouldn't occur otherwise.

But in the case of the HPV vaccine, the gold standard was set aside. In four of the five trials conducted by Merck and reviewed by the FDA, placebos to which Gardasil was compared contained an adjuvant, "a substance which enhances the body's immune response to an antigen." According to one of the trial publications, most of the Gardasil® trial placebos actually contained an "amorphous aluminium hydroxyphosphate sulfate adjuvant . . . and was visually indistinguishable from vaccine."

So although the majority of the placebo treatments in the Gardasil® trials did not include Gardasil® virus-like particles or VLPs, they were by no means inert. In control populations representing nearly 95 percent of all "placebo" recipients, the study subjects received a formulation that actually included an immunologically active (and potentially harmful) aluminum adjuvant.

In the fifth trial, the "placebo" was actually what's called a carrier solution, meaning it contained all the ingredients of the vaccine except the viral particles and aluminum. These ingredients included "yeast protein, sodium chloride [table salt], L-histidine [an amino acid], polysorbate 80 [an emulsifier], sodium borate, and water for injection." At least one of these chemicals, sodium borate, is a chemically reactive toxin, one that has many industrial uses as an active ingredient. Sodium borate has been used as a replacement for mercury in gold mining, an insecticide and fungicide, and a food additive that is now banned in the United States.

But even without a true placebo to measure against, the results were concerning. The vast majority of the Gardasil® (81%) and aluminum-adjuvant (75%) groups reported some kind of adverse event, most of which involved some kind of pain. By contrast, less than half of the carrier-solution group (45%) reported an adverse event. This pattern continues in almost all of the individual categories, with the Gardasil® group showing the largest rate of local reactions, followed closely by the aluminum-adjuvant group, and then with a clear drop off in the frequency of adverse events in the carrier-solution group. On a retrospective basis, all but one of the reduced risks for the carrier-solution group were statistically significant.

In the carrier-solution group, not a single recipient chose to drop out of the trial—often a sign of side effects. But there were three discontinuations after two weeks due to deaths in the Gardasil® group and one such death in the aluminum-adjuvant groups, whereas there were zero deaths at any point in the carrier-solution group. Seven discontinuations (four in the Gardasil® group and three in the aluminum-adjuvant group) were due to other severe adverse events. These are obviously small numbers; the reviewers dismissed the deaths as unrelated to vaccination.

As a result, the FDA approved Gardasil® without any idea of its real risks and still today is not in a position to say whether Gardasil® is safe *or* effective. This approach is symptomatic of the government's casual attitude toward vaccination-safety studies in general. There are numerous examples of other vaccine trials where the "placebo" results measured little to do with safety: the Menactra® vaccine trial compared the meningitis vaccine with another, previously approved, meningitis vaccine, Menomune®; similarly, the new high-tech hepatitis B vaccines were only tested for safety against the older hepatitis B vaccines that didn't use recombinant DNA technology.

In 2014, Canadian researchers, confirming studies in the US, found that the MMRV (measles, mumps, rubella, and chicken pox vaccines combined shot) in use there caused twice as many febrile seizures seven to ten days later as getting the MMR and chicken pox vaccines in separate shots. The idea of comparing the combined vaccine to a placebo never seemed to occur to the researchers.

Beyond these poorly designed individual-safety studies, the obvious issue of the expanding vaccine schedule is never even considered: When new vaccines are put on the schedule, they aren't tested against the rest of the vaccines children already get to see if interactions are a problem. And, of course, the most important safety study of all–testing total-health outcomes in vaccinated versus never-vaccinated children–remains suspiciously undone.

CHAPTER 7

THE LIVE-VIRUS VACCINES

- Mumps
- Measles
- Rubella
- Chicken pox

THE FOUR VACCINES IN THIS CATEGORY ARE PRODUCED BY WEAKENING BUT NOT KILLING—the technical word is *attenuating*—the viruses that produce the disease.

Three of these live-virus vaccines—mumps, measles, and rubella—are available in the United States only as a combination shot; the MMR vaccine combines those three into one shot, and the MMRV vaccine adds chicken pox (the V is for varicella, the medical name for the chicken pox virus).

The CDC recommends the MMR and the chicken pox vaccines at twelve to fifteen months, with boosters at age four to six years.

Mumps, measles, chicken pox, and rubella—better known as the German or three-day measles—need little introduction, at least for baby boomers. For centuries, they were common and even expected illnesses of childhood, with few complications in the developed world where good nutrition and sanitation prevail.

But you'd never know it from Merck's official product label for the M-M-R® II: "Measles, mumps, and rubella are three common childhood diseases . . . that may be associated with serious complications and/or death. For example, pneumonia and encephalitis are caused by measles. Mumps is associated with aseptic meningitis, deafness and orchitis (swollen testicles); and rubella during pregnancy may cause congenital rubella syndrome in the infants of infected mothers."

Rubella is, in fact, a special case—while not dangerous to children, it can be damaging and even deadly to a fetus. If a pregnant woman contracts rubella, the child can be stillborn or suffer birth defects ranging from deafness to cataracts to heart defects to intellectual disability. Because the rubella vaccine is not currently available as a separate injection in the United States, this may complicate the decision for many parents about whether their child should get the MMR.

That is not the only complication when considering the MMR and chicken pox vaccines.

- Many parents believe the MMR vaccination triggered their child's autistic regression, bowel problems, autoimmune disorders, and other chronic health conditions. In 2014, a CDC scientist admitted he and his colleagues failed to report evidence that giving the MMR to black males under thirty-six months of age increased the risk of autism.

- According to a whistleblower lawsuit filed by two former Merck scientists, the mumps portion of the vaccine is significantly less effective than claimed. This may be creating a dangerous situation if outbreaks occur and males catch the disease after puberty. At that point, mumps can lead to sterility in males.

- There is strong evidence that the chicken pox vaccine has increased the prevalence of shingles—trading a mostly trivial manifestation of the virus early in life for an excruciating and sometimes fatal one later on, and boosting the market for a shingles vaccine made by the same company!

- The rubella portion of the MMR is derived from cell lines originally prepared from tissues of aborted fetuses (as is the chicken pox vaccine, two vaccines against hepatitis A, and one each against polio, rabies, and smallpox). This creates an ethical problem for some parents, although the Vatican gave

Catholics a reluctant OK to use such vaccines. Beyond that is the issue of whether injected, human DNA could be dangerous and even a factor in the rise of autism.

Mumps Vaccine

Mumps, a viral infection whose characteristic sign is swollen salivary glands that puff up the cheeks and neck, is an ancient disease spread by coughing and sneezing. Hippocrates, the father of Western medicine, described it in the fifth century BC: "Swellings appeared about the ears, in many on either side, and in the greatest number on both sides, being unaccompanied by fever so as to confine the patient to bed; in all cases they disappeared without giving trouble." But in young men, "inflammations with pain seized sometimes one of the testicles, and sometimes both; some of these were accompanied with fever and some not; the greater part of these were attended with much suffering."

This description captures the two sides of mumps: in childhood, it generally passes without problems, causing swollen glands and a few days out of school, but in males who have reached puberty, it can be much worse and even lead to sterility.

Several different varieties of the mumps vaccine have been developed and sold since the vaccine was invented in the 1950s. These include the Urabe strain from Japan, the Leningrad-3 strain from Russia, and the Rubini strain from Switzerland. The current version of the mumps vaccine sold in the US was created by Maurice Hilleman, a Merck scientist who took a swab of the virus from his daughter Jeryl Lynn's throat in 1963 when she came down with the mumps. After attenuation, a "Jeryl Lynn strain" was approved for use in 1967 and first combined into the mumps-measles-rubella shot in 1971.

The mumps portion of the MMR has always proven to be the most troublesome for vaccine makers to get right. The Urabe strain has had a history of safety problems and soon in its commercial release led to cases of aseptic meningitis in Canada. Despite clear evidence of the problem in that country, it was the strain first used in the MMR in England and Europe.

This illustrates the tradeoff between reactogenic vaccines, which created strong immune responses that could lead to greater complications, and vaccines based on safer strains that generated fewer adverse reactions but were more likely to fail in the field. In all of these products, the vaccine strain is chasing a moving target, the wild strain in circulation, which may or may not benefit from protection with administration of the vaccine strain, Jeryl Lynn, Urabe, or otherwise. Some strains, like the Urabe, have a worse safety record; other strains, like Jeryl Lynn, have been shown to create less effective immune reactions.

Now, according to the authoritative medical manual, *Vaccines*, "mumps is making a comeback in nearly all countries where the disease had once been under control, and as seen in the US, cases of this historically childhood disease now predominantly occur in young adults." The outbreaks are occurring in fully vaccinated populations, and waning immunity is clearly implicated.

In May 2014, the *Akron Beacon Journal* reported a "growing number of mumps cases in central Ohio, where 339 people had confirmed cases of the disease as of Friday. Nearly two hundred of the cases have been linked to Ohio State University." Most had been vaccinated, the newspaper reported. In 2013 another mini-outbreak occurred in the South Atlantic, mostly in Virginia and Maryland.

But why is this happening, more than forty years after the vaccine began cutting the rate of mumps infection? After decades of passing the virus through the original strain, it appears the vaccine has lost much of its original effectiveness—a fact the manufacturer may have been hiding for years. In 2012, two Merck scientists filed a whistleblower lawsuit. The scientists say they witnessed a supervisor manually changing test results that showed the vaccine wasn't working, hurriedly destroying garbage bags full of evidence to keep the fraud from being exposed, and lying to FDA regulators who came to the lab after being alerted by the whistleblowers.

The alleged fraud occurred because, in order to maintain its license for the mumps-measles-rubella vaccine, known as the M-M-R® II, Merck needed to show that its Jeryl Lynn strain of the mumps vaccine was still as potent as when originally approved in 1967 as a single vaccine, able to induce immunity in 95 percent of those vaccinated. That number, according to vaccine authorities, is crucial because it leads to "herd immunity"—a form of immunity that occurs when enough of the population is immunized to protect against outbreaks even among unvaccinated people.

Reward Factors

Question 1: How bad is the disease?

The CDC says mumps is "usually a mild viral disease" but that one in twenty thousand children who got the mumps became deaf as a result. While brain inflammation (encephalitis) was a rare result of mumps (one in five hundred cases), it was still the leading cause of viral encephalitis. Pre-vaccine, children were usually between five and nine years old when they were infected—a number that crept up as vaccine coverage increased. That led to more serious problems: In males past puberty, swelling of the testicles occurred in 37 percent of cases, and women who caught mumps in the first trimester of pregnancy had a higher miscarriage rate.

Score: +1

Question 2: Does getting the vaccine help protect others from getting the same illness?

While the vaccine initially appeared to be effective in preventing the spread of the disease, the same claim can no longer be made as confidently. Resurgent outbreaks triggered more than 6,500 cases in college students in 2006 and more than 3,400 among observant Jews in 2009-2010. Most of the college students had been vaccinated but clearly were capable of catching mumps and passing it on to someone else. The former Merck scientists who have described fraud in the company's internal testing suggest that the success rate is far lower than the 95 percent the company claims.

Score: +4

Question 3: What is the risk of infection?

Mumps spreads like the common cold and is easily caught, although in many cases there is no apparent sign of infection. Herd immunity appears to have taken hold, but since vaccine failure has become so common, periodic cycles of mumps outbreaks, almost entirely among those previously vaccinated, have become a cyclical occurrence with outbreaks every three to four years.

Score: +1

Question 4: How well does the vaccine work?

Not at all well, according to the whistleblower lawsuit and the evidence of thousands of infections over the past several years, most in vaccinated individuals. The mumps vaccine may be the least effective of all vaccines.

Score: +1

Risk Factors for all three components

Question 1: What are the vaccine's side effects?

Most data of adverse events from mumps vaccines are derived from the Jeryl Lynn strain in the reactogenic M-M-R® II product, the only MMR vaccine licensed in the United States.

"The risk of MMR vaccine causing serious harm, or death, is extremely small," according to the CDC Vaccine Information Statement. Mild problems, according to the VIS, include fever in as many as one in six people, mild rash in one out of twenty, and swelling of glands in the cheek or neck in about one in seventy-five.

Moderate problems include fever-induced seizures in 1 out of 3,000; temporary pain and joint stiffness in 1 out of 4, mostly in teenage or adult women; transient low-platelet count, which can trigger a bleeding disorder, in 1 in 30,000.

Severe problems, which the CDC calls "very rare," include allergic reaction, occurring in fewer than 1 in a million; deafness; "long-term seizures, coma, or lowered consciousness"; and permanent brain damage (in so few cases that the CDC says it is hard to know if the vaccine caused them).

The statement makes no mention of the significant risk to older males if they catch mumps because the vaccine efficacy is too low or wears off.

Score: -1

Question 2: What are the risks of chronic/severe illness and death?

The MMR vaccine is probably the most controversial drug in the public debate over autism. Although mainstream scientists claim "study after study" refutes any association, thousands of parents say they have witnessed their children become ill and regress immediately after vaccination. The designs of the studies purporting to demonstrate the safety of mumps and MMR vaccines have come under withering criticism by vaccine-safety organizations.

"Kapoore," a commenter on our blog, said: "I wish I had not given my daughter the MMR and instead she had gotten the measles. . . . As a result of the MMR she developed ataxia (loss of muscle control), couldn't hold a pencil, ended up with an autoimmune disease, and was sick for twenty years with immune failure. I had the measles and it lasted two weeks."

A blogger at Livingwhole.org made the same point in June 2014 in a post titled, "Measles Shmeasles":

> So far, in 2014 there have been 288 cases of measles, no cases of encephalitis, and no death. In 2013 there were 189 cases of measles, no encephalitis and no death. In 2012 there were 54 cases of measles, no encephalitis, and no death. In 2011, there were 22 cases of measles, and you guessed it . . . no encephalitis, and no death. I could go on, but you get the point. By and large, measles is unpleasant, not deadly.
>
> In comparison, the same cannot be said for the MMR vaccine. As of March 1, 2012 there were 842 serious injuries following the MMR vaccine and 56 deaths. Since 1990 there have been more than 6,058 serious adverse events reported to the Vaccine Adverse Events Reporting System (VAERS). What's even more sad is that only 1–10% of cases are actually reported on this database.

Furthermore, the rubella component of the vaccine has a clear association with arthritis.

Score: -4

Question 3: What are the consequences of using the vaccine in combination with other vaccines?

When the vaccine is given as part of ProQuad®, the risk of febrile seizures doubles. The CDC says the seizures are not dangerous, but it's hard to see why any parent would want to take that risk just for the "convenience" of a four-in-one shot.

Because the measles, mumps, and rubella vaccine is only available in combination shots, the only way to receive it is with at least two other vaccines. That means they interact with each other in ways that don't occur when children catch these diseases at different times—or, for that matter, if the vaccines were spaced far enough apart to avoid the problem, which is called viral interference.

Once again, public health officials say that in the vaccine formulation, there's no problem. But there are some worrisome signs, both from studies of the vaccines and from real-world experience when children catch more than one of the diseases at the same time.

One example: Studies in the UK and Iceland showed that when mumps and measles epidemics hit these populations in the same year, the risk of inflammatory bowel disease—often seen in autistic children—spiked.

In a 1979 report, "Viral Exposure and Autism," in the *American Journal of Epidemiology,* the authors looked at whether certain viruses, either in pregnancy or in infancy, can be linked to autism.

"The data indicates that total autistic symptomatology seems to be associated with prenatal viral experience with measles and mumps and with infancy illness or exposure to mumps and chickenpox."

While they're talking about the "wild" viral infection in these studies, not vaccines, any association between autism and the same viruses now given in combination shots to babies ought to raise alarms. There's also how early the shots are given—few kids ever get the actual diseases at age one, when the vaccine is recommended; they're protected by the immunity from their mother's antibodies to the diseases.

The measles vaccine, ironically, weakened the immunity against measles that mothers pass on to their children. Because vaccinated mothers didn't catch the actual disease themselves in childhood, their antibodies are not as effective. For that reason, the vaccine recommendation was moved closer to birth for infants—from 15 months to 12–15 months. That in turn may increase the risk to the infant.

Dr. Jeff Bradstreet, a family practitioner in Florida who has treated several thousand autistic children, warns that younger children are more vulnerable because their immune and neurological systems are immature.

"There's definitely been an association of kids getting MMR at twelve months and crashing" with autism and other health problems, Bradstreet said.

That's why some critics believe the shots should be given separately, perhaps a year apart. Unfortunately, that's not an option in the United States.

Score: -4

Question 4: Are there ways to protect against the disease without getting the vaccine?

Before vaccination, these were diseases almost every child caught. Keeping a child at home and away from children known to be infected is the best way to avoid them. But exposing a child at an early age is often a safe path to lifelong immunity.

Score: 0

Overall Reward-Risk Rating: -2

The Big Picture: Making Mild Illnesses Dangerous

In our pill-popping culture, the word "medicine" has lost the meaning of "healing profession" and become a synonym for pharmaceuticals.

But in the case of mumps and several other childhood illnesses, letting nature take her course may be preferrable.

Mumps is generally a harmless childhood disease but very risky and painful when infection comes later, a consequence for which the vaccine is responsible.

What's more, the vaccine itself has been a big problem. Early vaccines using the Urabe strain often caused adverse reactions and were pulled. SmithKline Beecham's Pluserix brand, which contained the Urabe mumps strain, was first introduced in 1986 in Canada and then abruptly pulled from the market only two years later. Amazingly, Pluserix was then introduced into the UK market in the same year in 1988, only to be withdrawn due to adverse events in 1991. Meanwhile, both Japan and New Zealand withdrew Urabe strain versions of MMR in 1992.

The chicken pox vaccine has led to another problem—a rise in shingles, the truly dangerous form of the disease. Before the chicken pox vaccine became ubiquitous, people who had the illness as a child got an immunological "bump" by being exposed to an active case of chicken pox. This tune-up helped remind the immune system to recognize the virus that the body was already harboring and reduce shingles attacks.

But with the opportunity to encounter chicken pox all but gone, more shingles cases are occurring, and in younger people. (The chicken pox vaccine manufacturer, Merck, is making millions selling a new shingles vaccine called Zostavax®. By 2013, Zostavax® sales had risen from zero to $758 million annually in just eight years.)

Other common illnesses may have played complicated but crucial roles in the immune system. Scientists recently reported they were able to rid a patient of a type of cancer called multiple myeloma by injecting her with a massive dose of the measles vaccine. Other signs that standard childhood diseases can prep the body to ward off truly serious threats: less cancer of the ovaries in women who had childhood mumps, remissions in leukemia and lymphoma cases during measles and rubella infections, and deliberate measles infections to battle pediatric nephrotic syndrome, a serious kidney condition.

Even poliovirus may have its purpose: In 2011, doctors infused a genetically altered poliovirus into a twenty-year-old nursing student's brain tumor, which at the time was the size of a tennis ball.

Two years later, she is cancer free, and doctors say the prospect of using viruses against cancer is intriguing.

None of this comes as news to old-line pediatricians like Harold Buttram, who wrote that "the cellular immune system, lacking former challenges of the so-called 'minor childhood diseases' of former times (measles, mumps, chickenpox, and rubella) may be going through the process of atrophy of disuse, also being further compromised by the immunosuppressant effects of combination-viral vaccines. . . . Only these four [childhood illnesses] significantly challenged and therefore strengthened the immunity of the epithelial and endothelial tissues of the body and their associated organs."

And now they can be wiped out in just one shot.

Measles Vaccine

Measles is a highly contagious airborne virus, communicable by simply walking by an infected person in an airport or drugstore. It has been described in medical literature since the Middle Ages and is related to a disease of cattle called rinderpest, which probably made the jump to humans when we began domesticating animals.

Much of the recent publicity about measles reflects a small increase in US cases in the past few years—usually overseas travelers becoming infected and then spreading the illness in small pockets that generate alarmist headlines.

In the spring of 2014, a news outlet in suburban Washington, under a large banner titled "Health Warning," reported public health workers "are informing people who were at various locations . . . that they may have been exposed to a person with measles. Northern Virginia area health officials are mounting a coordinated effort to identify people who may have been exposed."

The idea that measles is highly infectious is certainly true; the claim that it is a health emergency is not. For generations, measles was considered a rite of passage for children, with little risk of complications and the reward of lifetime immunity. A doll from 1958 named Hedda Gets Better has two faces on opposite sides of her head, one with the familiar measles spots and the other blemish-free for the child to turn around and be reminded that the disease clears up.

Almost always in the US and other developed countries, children do get better. Within ten to fourteen days of exposure, the patient develops a fever, cough, and reddish eyes, followed by a rash that begins in the mouth and on the head and spreads to the rest of the body. Fever up to 105 degrees and itching can make the child quite uncomfortable for several days. Sometimes, ear infections or pneumonia can occur, which are treatable by antibiotics.

Rarely, severe complications ensue—brain inflammation, called encephalitis, and pneumonia that can be life-threatening. The CDC claims that one in a thousand who catch the measles dies, but the historic record shows that death rates from measles had fallen essentially to zero before the vaccine came along. In England and Wales, deaths of those under fifteen dropped from 1,100 in the middle 1800s to nearly zero just before the vaccine was given; a similar trajectory occurred in the United States.

The first vaccine was licensed in 1963, meaning that most adults in their mid-fifties and older have had the illness. Many of them look on with amazement at the fear the illness engenders. The impact of the vaccine was less about saving lives than keeping kids in school.

MEASLES INCIDENCE AND MORTALITY IN THE 20TH CENTURY

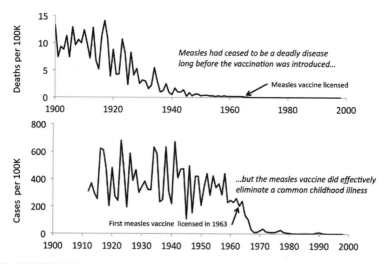

Reward Factors

Question 1: How bad is the disease?

In its Vaccine Information Statement, the CDC warns measles "can lead to ear infection, pneumonia, seizures (jerking and staring), brain damage, and death." These risks are negligible in developed countries, however.

Score: +3

Question 2: Does getting the vaccine help protect others from getting the same illness?

Yes. Measles spreads through respiratory droplets from sneezing and coughing and can linger on contaminated surfaces for several hours. It is hard to avoid: Between half a million to a million cases were reported each year in the late 1950s; that number plunged precipitously to less than fifty thousand by the late 1950s and now totals fewer than five hundred. Because it is a live virus, the vaccine itself can spread measles.

Score: +4

Question 3: What is the risk of infection?

Very low today. The few hundred cases of measles reported in the United States each year, out of four million births, mean the chance of a child catching it are negligible, despite the scary headlines.

Score: 0

Question 4: How well does the vaccine work?

The measles component of the MMR vaccine appears to be effective, although some cases have occurred in vaccinated individuals. In about 5 percent of cases, the vaccine simply fails to take. The booster shot before kindergarten is intended to induce immunity in those kids by giving it again to every child. An option we'll discuss in Part 3 is to check blood titers before the second shot is due; if immunity is indicated, the second shot is not necessary.

Score: +4

Risk Factors (see mumps)

Question 1: What are the vaccine's side effects?

Score: -1

Question 2: What are the risks of chronic/severe illness and death?

Score: -4

Question 3: What are the consequences of using the vaccine in combination with other vaccines?

Score: -4

Question 4: Are there ways to protect against the disease without getting the vaccine?

Score: 0

Overall Reward-Risk Rating: 2

The Big Picture: When Food Is the Best Medicine

Good nutrition trumps vaccination as a health measure. The death rate from most diseases for which vaccines have been developed plummeted well before the introduction of vaccines. Measles can, in rare cases, cause problems in those infected, but these are far greater issues in less developed regions with poor nutrition. Vitamin A deficiency has been associated with measles problems, but when a child is well nourished and cared for, measles is generally harmless.

The World Health Organization says 122,000 people die globally from measles every year, almost none of them in the United States.

The WHO notes: "Severe measles is more likely among poorly nourished young children, especially those with insufficient vitamin A, or whose immune systems have been weakened by HIV/AIDS or other diseases. . . . As high as 10% of measles cases result in death among populations with high levels of malnutrition and a lack of adequate health care. . . . More than 95% of measles deaths occur in countries with low per capita incomes and weak health infrastructures. . . . Overcrowding in residential camps greatly increases the risk of infection."

Measles is emblematic of other illnesses that are no threat in the developed world but still pursued zealously by public health officials in this country. Rotavirus is also a disease of poor nutrition and sanitation. As many as 450,000 children around the world died of the diarrheal disease before the vaccination was launched in 1998, but a miniscule fraction died in the United States. As long as a child is well nourished and hydrated, rotavirus constitutes little threat. Nonetheless, the CDC recommended universal vaccination for children in 1998; the shot turned out to cause a serious bowel problem that led to deaths. Two new vaccines have led to similar reports.

Rubella Vaccine

In Agatha Christie's 1962 mystery, *The Mirror Crack'd From Side To Side* (warning: spoiler alert), an actress takes revenge on a devoted fan who accidentally infected her with rubella. The actress was pregnant, and the fetus developed congenital rubella syndrome (CRS). The plot was probably based on the real-life saga of actress Gene Tierney; she was pregnant with her first daughter when infected in 1943 by a Marine who snuck out of quarantine to meet her. The daughter was born intellectually disabled, and Tierney, who was already dealing with mental health issues, was devastated; it could be said that neither ever recovered.

While measles and mumps are not typically serious diseases, rubella is a different and unusual story. At first blush, rubella seems to be the mildest: For most children, it is not just an innocous disease but one that many parents don't even notice, except for the presence of a rash.

It took a stroke of fate for doctors to realize that in the case of pregnancy, the outcome could be dire. In 1940, a particularly severe outbreak of German measles hit army training camps in Australia, and a large number of troops brought it home and infected their wives. The next year, an ophthalmologist in Sydney, Australia, Dr. Norman McAlister Gregg, noticed he was being referred an unusual number of infants with congenital cataracts. Some also had serious heart problems. Gregg checked with colleagues in New South Wales and Victoria and soon had compiled seventy-eight such cases. In sixty-eight of them, he realized, the mothers reported having had German measles either right before or very early in pregnancy. Other such cases cases showed a high rate of deafness.

The previously unsuspected link between rubella in the pregnant mother and a whole host of birth defects was soon confirmed by retrospective studies that found "deaf-mutism" in babies soared after rubella epidemics hit Australia. The same pattern was recognized in the United States and Europe as well.

Sceintists began searching in earnest for rubella treatments, the first of which were called gamma globulin—sets of antibodies pooled with human blood. By the 1960s, these products were used on a large scale and considered effective (though we have raised the possibilty that, because they were preserved with mercury, they ultimately made CRS a more damaging disease than it already was, including cases of autism).

In 1969, the rubella vaccine was introduced based on the identification of the virus seven years earlier. Congenital rubella disappeared in the United States, although it persists around the world.

To our minds, rubella vaccination is perhaps the single most valuable childhood immunization from a public health perspective. It prevents a disease that can permanently damage a fetus and even be fatal. Thus the case for universal coverage with rubella vaccinations is strong, even though the real risk of the disease is not to the children who receive the vaccine.

As it is, the only way to provide protection to pregnant women is to get the shot as part of the MMR vaccine, recommended starting at age one and again before kindergarten, or as ProQuad®. This creates a tough choice for parents, which we will take up in Part 3.

Reward Factors

Question 1: How bad is the disease?

Colloquially known as German measles, rubella is just another child-hood disease when it strikes infants and children, but it is dangerous for the developing fetus. Congenital rubella syndrome can occur when a pregnant woman contracts the disease during or just before her first trimester. Problems are unlikely if she contracts the disease after twenty weeks.

Score: +2

Question 2: Does getting the vaccine help protect others from getting the same illness?

Yes, universal adoption of the vaccine has wiped out rubella, and congenital rubella syndrome, in the United States. By contrast, during the last major epidemic, in 1964, twenty thousand infants were born with severe birth defects in the United States.

Score: +5

Question 3: What is the risk of infection?

US public health officials declared rubella eradicated in the United States in 2004, although cases continue to appear, especially in Hispanic people who have not been immunized. Traveling to areas where rubella still circulates—outside the Americas, according to the CDC—carries a risk of contracting the disease, and the center recommends that all travelers be vaccinated.

Score: 0

Question 4: How well does the vaccine work?

It appears to be the most effective vaccine in the MMR—the measles can spread even to vaccinated individuals, and the mumps portion appears very weak. By contrast, widespread rubella vaccination has nearly eliminated the virus from the United States.

Score: +4

Risk Factors (see mumps)

Question 1: What are the vaccine's side effects?

Score: -1

Question 2: What are the risks of chronic/severe illness and death?

Score: -4

Question 3: What are the consequences of using the vaccine in combination with other vaccines?

Score: -4

Question 4: Are there ways to protect against the disease without getting the vaccine?

Score: 0

Overall Reward-Risk Rating: 2

The Big Picture: When the Risk Is From Mother to Child

Rubella is the best example of the risk of passing on illness to a child. It's worth preventing, but even so, some of the steps taken to prevent it may have been misguided. And in general, the fear of infants catching illnesses from their mothers has led to a climate of fear and overprotection in obstetrics.

In our book, we noted that during the worldwide rubella outbreak in 1964, signs of autism first emerged as one of the outcomes of congenital rubella syndrome (CRS). We suggested that might be because a new gamma globulin treatment preserved with thimerosal was widely used.

A similar phenomenon has been identified with RhoGAM®, an injection given to pregnant women who are Rh negative in order to prevent Rh disease in their newborns. When a mother's blood type is negative and the developing baby's is positive, the shot stops the creation of antibodies to the Rh positive blood. It, too, was preserved with thimerosal (since removed), and several studies link RhoGAM® injections during pregnancy with autism.

Influenza vaccination for pregnant women—with shots still preserved with thimerosal—is another attempt to ward off complications for the fetus that, in our view, carries far more risk than reward.

The recommendation for a Tdap shot in pregnancy, to keep the mother (and other close contacts) from developing pertussis, is designed to "cocoon" the baby against the virus. But again, we worry that the risk of immune stimulation to the baby outweighs the risk of the disease itself.

Finally, universal hep B vaccination at birth—given the less-than-one-percent chance that a hep B-positive mother will infect her newborn (not the fetus)—takes things to absurdity.

Rubella is a real risk to a developing fetus, and the vaccination deserves consideration by parents as a contribution to public health. But the environment of fear it helped create in obstetric care isn't doing mothers, babies, or society in general any good.

Chicken pox Vaccine

Chicken pox is among the most innocuous of childhood illnesses, and the campaign to create a vaccine, have the government recommend it, and the states mandate it for school attendance is hard to take at face value.

Given how trivial the disease itself is, public health officials resorted to a kind of argument of convenience—parents, especially moms, would most likely miss work to stay home with a sick child. That costs the economy in lost wages and productivity. Therefore, the argument continues, it makes sense to vaccinate children, not so much for their sake as for society's. It is, essentially, a utilitarian economic decision masquerading as concern for children's health.

But like German measles, this relatively benign illness comes with a dangerous kicker. You've no doubt seen the ads about shingles that intone, "If you've had chickenpox, the virus that causes shingles is already inside you."

That's true—the chicken pox virus takes up residence in the peripheral nervous system, and when a person is under physical or even mental stress or other immune challenge, it can manifest as painful, persistent, and sometimes deadly shingles, characterized by a rash that follows one side of the nervous system, sometimes infecting the eye or other vital organs.

The irony here is that shingles has actually increased since the advent of the chicken pox vaccine. People who've had chicken pox and are subsequently exposed to active cases get an immune system "bump," a kind of immunological tune-up. It's no coincidence shingles cases have increased, and affected younger people, since the chicken pox vaccine became widespread.

The final irony is that the same company—Merck—that manufactures the chicken pox vaccine also makes the shingles vaccine, which is basically the same vaccine with about four times the amount of live-but-weakened chicken pox virus.

Reward Factors

Question 1: How bad is the disease?

Chicken pox is not a disease worth worrying about, despite the very few severe cases that are hyped to make it seem like a nightmare. The CDC warns that chickenpox "can lead to severe skin infection, scars, pneumonia, brain damage, or death." Such dire consequences are extremely rare, especially when children catch the illness at typical ages (peak incidence is five to nine years old); for the CDC to trumpet them in this distorted way suggests something skewed about its entire approach to illness—hyping the dangers from the infection, hiding the risks from the inoculation.

Score: +1

Question 2: Does getting the vaccine help protect others from getting the same illness?

Yes, if we're talking about the benign childhood illness. But it deprives those already infected with the immunological reminder that helps suppress shingles. Some parents hold "chicken pox parties" when a child in the neighborhood shows signs of it, trying to expose their children and get the disease out of the way at a young age. This maternal wisdom is treated as dangerous nonsense by the current crop of vaccine zealots pushing every vaccine they can invent and market.

Score: 0

Question 3: What is the risk of infection?

Low in the United States now. Many developed countries, such as Great Britain, don't require the vaccine, which might make it easier to find chicken pox parties outside the United States.

Score: +1

Question 4: How well does the vaccine work?

The chicken pox vaccine appears to have created herd immunity. But it also takes two vaccinations. The chicken pox vaccine was first licensed for children over twelve months of age in 1995, but a study showed that among adolescents given one shot, only 79 percent had "seroconverted," with sufficient antibodies to fight an actual infection.

In 2006, a booster shot was recommended for children ages four to six years.

Score: +4

Risk Factors

Question 1: What are the vaccine's side effects?

The CDC says mild side effects include soreness or swelling at the injection site in 1 out of 5 children and up to 1 in 3 adolescents, fever in 1 out of 10 or fewer, and mild rash up to a month later in 1 in 25. The latter individuals may be infectious, the CDC notes, but actual transmission is rare.

Moderate problems include seizure due to fever, which the CDC says is very rare. Severe problems include pneumonia, also very rare, as well as severe brain reactions and low blood count, which are so rare it's not clear whether the vaccine actually causes them.

If you get the MMRV shot, the CDC reports rash and fever are more common after the first dose of the MMRV vaccine compared to the chicken pox shot alone, and seizures caused by fever are also more common, usually five to twelve days after the shot.

Score: -1

Question 2: What are the risks of chronic/severe illness and death?

Any live-virus vaccine carries the risk of triggering the disease it is designed to prevent, and even being infectious for a period of time after the shot.

Although the MMR vaccine is the live-virus shot most often associated with the onset of autism by parents, the chicken pox vaccine also figures in some accounts. We've written about the case of Ryan Boe in Olympia, Washington, who at age eighteen months got four shots at one office visit, including the chicken pox vaccine. (Ryan got his MMR shot two months earlier.) "Before we could leave the office he had an allergic reaction where he broke out in hives on his legs where they'd given him the shots," Ryan's mother, Lisa, recalls about that day, November 3, 2003. "And then I think it was about two or three hours later after leaving the doctor's office that he started running a fever."

Within a month, his loss of expression and connection had become obvious. An autism diagnosis followed.

Score: -4

Question 3: What are the consequences of using the vaccine in combination with other vaccines?

In general, as Ryan Boe's experience demonstrates, it's not a good idea to get a live-virus shot in combination with multiple other vaccines, so it just makes sense to avoid the chicken pox shot at the same visit as the MMR, or live-virus influenza or rotavirus vaccination.

Score: -4

Question 4: Are there ways to protect against the disease without getting the vaccine?

The usual precautions of avoiding sick kids, washing hands, and disinfecting common surfaces. But if a child is unvaccinated and exposed to someone with chicken pox, they are likely to become infected. Consider it exercise for the developing immune system.

Score: 0

OVERALL RISK-REWARD SCORE: -5

The Big Picture: Facing the Problem of Viral Interference

Live-virus vaccines are inherently dangerous for the simple fact that the viruses are *alive*—attenuated, yes, but still capable of interaction, replication, and persistence. The message from multiple studies seems to be the same—combining multiple live viruses in one shot, or giving them at the same time in separate shots, is a dangerous thing to do. And it's not even necessary. When the MMRV vaccine—the MMR vaccine with chicken pox (varicella) vaccine added—was introduced as ProQuad®, the amount of weakened chicken pox virus required to trigger an immune reaction was substantially higher than in the chicken pox vaccine alone. Why? Because putting so many different viruses into a single vaccine created a problem of interference in the immune system. This has been an issue in other components of ProQuad® as well.

In 2005, Merck reported that "measles-like rash and fever during days 5–12 were more common after the first dose of MMRV [ProQuad]" than after the MMR vaccine and Varivax® given separately. The difference was substantial—5.9 percent who got the MMRV vaccine had the rash and 27.7 percent had fever, compared to 1.9 percent with rash and 18.7 percent fever after getting separate shots.

The issue arose again in 2004, before the quadruple vaccine was approved. According to notes of a CDC meeting, Merck's Dr. Florian Schodel "confirmed the possibility that the chickenpox virus component of ProQuad was causing a local immune suppression and an increase in measles virus replication. . . . The current hypothesis is that the varicella and measles virus are co-infecting the same or proximate areas of the body and engaging in a specific interaction, but how that works is as yet unknown." *"How that works is as yet unknown"* should cause every parent to remain concerned, not just about the quadruple vaccine but any combination of live viruses.

A 1973 study looked at subacute sclerosing panencephalitis (SSPE), a delayed and often deadly brain infection that occurs in a small percentage of children who get measles, and found what we view as a similar red flag.

The authors, led by Roger Detels of the Division of Epidemiology at the UCLA School of Public Health, wanted to identify risk factors for developing the subsequent brain infection. The study matched thirty-eight children who had SSPE with thirty-eight who did not and reported: "Among the 38 matched pairs, 6 patients had had chickenpox six months or less before measles. . . . This sequence did not occur among controls."

This amounts to a "significant excess of chickenpox associated with measles in SSPE patients," the study concluded. "While this occurred in only six instances it is of note because of the relatively early age of clinical measles in patients versus controls, decreasing the likelihood of this sequence."

The message is clear: Getting viruses close together at young ages increases the risk of brain damage. Yet that is the way the CDC childhood immunization schedule is designed and arranged—maybe the right word is *deranged*.

CHAPTER 8

THE INFLUENZA VACCINE

WHY WOULD YOU EVER GET AN INFLUENZA VACCINE, commonly known as a flu shot? Supposedly, you'd do it for all kinds of reasons—to protect children, pregnant women, ill people, and old people, and to keep from feeling like death warmed over yourself or actually dying. How could anyone—how could *you*—resist?

You could resist for plenty of reasons. The influenza vaccine is unique among childhood vaccines in several ways, all of them concerning. First, it is routinely recommended for both children and adults—an annual shot starting at six months and continuing throughout life. It is the one annual lifetime vaccine, and signs of serious, adverse events appear at every age.

Second, it is recommended for all pregnant women, the only such vaccine besides the Tdap. Yet research suggests that stimulating the immune system during pregnancy—even artificially, with a vaccine—is dangerous for the developing fetus.

And influenza vaccine is unique for one more reason—despite the fact that the CDC and the American Academy of Pediatrics recommended in 1999 that the organic-mercury preservative called thimerosal be phased out of all shots given to children, multidose, inactivated-influenza vaccines still contain it.

Why on Earth would anyone expose pregnant women and infants to a neurotoxin, especially one as bad as mercury, in this supposedly enlightened day and age? This appears to be motivated by public health officials' concerns that if a new epidemic of influenza hit, they would need to be able to use multidose packages to enhance the available vaccine supply and protect more of the population. Some states have banned thimerosal, only to have their health department turn right around and invoke "emergency" exemptions that allow its continued use during that year's flu season.

Keeping thimerosal in influenza vaccines in the United States also makes it easier for other countries to justify its use in a wide range of vaccinations. How bad can it be, if the United States won't ban it? (The United Nations even hammered out a new agreement to reduce mercury exposure worldwide that specifically exempted mercury-containing vaccines, the most potent form of exposure.)

Whatever the rationale, the idea that an infant or fetus can still be exposed to mercury via a vaccine is unconscionable. If you take nothing else from *Vaccines 2.0*, we urge you never to let yourself or your child get a mercury-containing shot and to discourage people you care about from doing the same.

All in all, this vaccine reminds us of the big league baseball scout sent to review a supposedly promising minor league player. His succinct report: "Although he can't hit or throw, at least he cannot catch."

Peter Doshi, a scientist at Johns Hopkins University, put it this way in 2013: "The vaccine may be less beneficial and less safe than has been claimed, and the threat of influenza seems to be overstated. For most people, and possibly most doctors, officials need only claim that vaccines save lives, and it is assumed there must be solid research behind it."

That hasn't stopped the push for the annual flu shot—posters all over grocery stores, relentless warnings in the media about the approach of flu season, and ultimatums by health-care employers. "Get vaccinated or get out" is the mantra of much of modern medicine.

Professor Doshi's own employer, Johns Hopkins, has such a policy: "The mandatory influenza vaccination program applies to all individuals, employees, faculty, staff, residents and fellows, temporary workers, trainees, volunteers, students, vendors and voluntary medical staff, regardless of employer, who provide services to patients or work in patient care. . . ."

In support of such a broad policy, Johns Hopkins claims, "each year, approximately 36,000 people die and 226,000 are hospitalized due to the flu. These are preventable deaths."

But those figures, like other statistics ginned up to pave the way for dubious mass vaccination campaigns such as hep B vaccination at birth, are seriously overstated, the kind of thing Doshi means when he says doctors assume "there must be solid research" behind such claims.

There isn't. According to the respected Cochrane Collaboration, influenza is a relatively small portion of flu-like illnesses. The group reviewed flu studies and found that 7 percent of the population get flu-like symptoms in any given year; the proportion that's actually influenza is just 7 percent *of that*, or not quite half a percent of the population. The rest is the common cold, respiratory syncytial viruses, stomach bugs, and other ailments that people pass off as "the flu."

The evidence, Cochrane reported, "points to influenza being a relatively rare cause of influenza-like illness and a relatively rare disease. It follows that vaccines may not be an appropriate intervention for either influenza or influenza-like illness."

It's worth pausing over that: "influenza being a relatively rare cause of influenza-like illness"! In other words, you may feel like you have influenza, but you probably don't. To know for sure, your doctor would need to take a nasal swab, which is rarely done because "the flu" is so often the presumptive diagnosis.

What's more, the influenza vaccine you get might not be helpful in preventing the strains circulating that year; a committee of scientists picks three or four strains to blend into one injection, and then drug makers ramp up production to try to get the vaccine into circulation in time. It's an educated guess, and like many guesses, it is often wrong.

In 1999, the CDC, the American Academy of Pediatrics, and the American Association of Family Medicine all recommended that thimerosal be removed from children's vaccines—at that point the DTaP, Hib, and hep B vaccines. Influenza vaccines were not broadly recommended except for some high-risk groups.

But as mercury was phased out of the other shots, broader coverage of mercury-containing influenza vaccines was phased in and now includes all pregnant women and everyone else, starting at age six months.

How does this jibe with the statement from the CDC and pediatricians in 2000 that urged, "continuation of the current policy of moving rapidly to vaccines which are free of thimerosal as a preservative"? It doesn't. The Wizard of Oz–like expectation that you pay no attention to their own statement points to the hubris behind the curtain of the vaccine establishment.

And the fact that influenza vaccines during pregnancy have not been adequately studied is no secret. It's right there on package inserts. Reads one: "Safety and effectiveness of Fluzone Quadrivalent have not been established in pregnant women or children less than 6 months of age."

In 2014, a CDC senior scientist named William W. Thompson, who led several important vaccine safety studies, made news when he said he would never let his pregnant wife get a thimerosal-containing shot.

We repeat, why would you ever get a flu shot?

There are six brands and two kinds of influenza vaccines on the market in the United States—live/attenuated virus and killed/inactivated virus. It is the killed-virus, multidose vials that have thimerosal.

Some of the vaccines are designed to protect against three strains of influenza, others against four. The nasal-spray vaccine, a live-virus formulation, is recommended for healthy children ages two through eight.

Otherwise, the CDC doesn't state a preference for which of the vaccines kids and pregnant women get—a profound moral failure, since a high percentage contain thimerosal. No one, least of all pregnant women and infants, should be exposed to that neurotoxic chemical.

Reward Factors

Question 1: How bad is the disease?

Influenza can be a miserable experience, but it's almost always survivable. The CDC clearly inflates the number of annual influenza deaths, to around thirty-six thousand a year, just as it did with hepatitis B in children when it was pushing to get that vaccine on the schedule. Their influenza figure includes pneumonia and other complications.

As you weigh the choice for your baby, know that there is some pediatric mortality from influenza: fewer than 100 cases nationally per year and usually in immunocompromised children. Having a healthy infant die from influenza is extraordinarily rare.

Score: +1

Question 2: Does getting the vaccine help protect others from getting the same illness?

Part of the rationale for giving the influenza vaccine to children is to protect the elderly, and there is a big push to get the elderly the shot on the theory that frail people with weakened immune systems are likelier to die from influenza. (There's a high-dose shot targeted at those sixty-five and older.) The Cochrane Collaboration says there's no evidence the shot reduces the mortality rate in the elderly.

Others suspect that at least part of the reason that more elderly die during flu season is from the shot itself. Adult children of aging parents often notice cognitive and general health decline in association with the annual influenza vaccine that so many senior-living centers require.

So the notion that you're giving your baby an influenza vaccine to protect Grandma is not a good argument. Is it really worth performing a risky procedure on an infant?

Yes, getting vaccinated can help, but the strains in the influenza vaccine must match the ones circulating that year. The live-virus nasal spray, because it sheds virus, could actually be a risk. Recipients are advised to stay away from immunocompromised individuals for several weeks. That's ironic, given that the shot is heavily marketed as protecting such people, and given that it's offered like candy in very public places such as grocery stores with very little warning to the immunocompromised.

Score: +2

Question 3: What is the risk of infection?

Influenza spreads easily through droplets. It's one of the more infectious diseases. A big concern of public health officials is when a mutant virus takes off from some remote location—say, avian flu, which originated in birds and was transmitted throughout Asia beginning in 2003. Or consider H1N1, which originated in pigs in Mexico. Again, the risk of catching influenza is slight and, in healthy people, survivable, while the vaccines crafted to subdue it are risky and not necessarily effective.

Score: +3

Question 4: How well does the vaccine work?

Often not very well. How many times have you heard people say, "I got the flu shot and then I got the flu"? In some cases, that may actually be side effects from the shot. But we have a friend who got the shot, got lab-tested influenza later that season, and was told by his doctor, "It would have been worse if you hadn't gotten the shot."

Score: +1

Risk Factors

Question 1: What are the vaccine's side effects?

We hear lots of horror stories about influenza vaccines. Lisa Marks-Smith, who lived in Cincinnati, suffered paralysis, severe neurological problems, and twenty-four days in the hospital—and got a substantial check from the Vaccine Injury Compensation Program that attests to the truth of her story. Desiree Jennings, a Washington Redskins cheerleader, developed a bizarre movement disorder right after getting the shot. She made her challenges public and was promptly attacked by Internet trolls claiming she made it all up.

With a billion and a half doses produced yearly, the influenza vaccine is far and away the most widely given vaccine. But with healthy adults the primary target, the adverse events rate is, not surprisingly, fairly low. Gayle DeLong's analysis of VAERS data found the vaccine-adverse-event rate per recipient is less than many other vaccines given exclusively to children.

Possible vaccine injuries are also harder to track, now that the influenza vaccine is given everywhere from grocery stores to kiosks in airports. (Save your receipt if you get an influenza vaccine in such places; it may be the only proof you have if you suffer a reaction and the company tries to deny it ever gave you the shot!) So these reported rates in many respects understate the risks.

Seen from a different perspective, because the influena vaccine is the most frequently given, there are also more adverse events entered into VAERS from these vaccines than any others. Gayle DeLong's analysis shows over 50,000 adverse events, nearly 2,400 of them life-threatening, including more than 1,100 deaths. Influenza deaths in children are generally less than one hundred a year. (And remember, the rate of reporting to VAERS reflects just a fraction of similar incidents.)

Internal CDC documents obtained by vaccine-safety advocate Brian Hooker and shared with the authors suggest other major problems may be lurking in the data, such as higher rates of Guillain-Barré syndrome, a paralytic disorder; Bell's palsy, which paralyzes facial muscles; seizures; and abnormal neurologic symptoms.

Score: -4

Question 2: What are the risks of chronic/severe illness and death?

In part because it is given so frequently, the influenza vaccine has the highest number of deaths reported in any category. Recovery from injuries caused by the influenza vaccine can take years, if they do not become permanent.

Score: -4

Question 3: What are the consequences of using the vaccine in combination with other vaccines?

It's often given alone to healthy adults. There's not a lot of good evidence of its interaction with other vaccines, but we suspect thimerosal—still in many of the vaccine doses given—causes problems when it interacts with live-virus vaccines and those containing aluminum.

In children, two doses of the flu shot are given starting at age six months, separated by at least a month, followed by one every year thereafter. At the six- and eighteen-month visits, this comes on top of other shots including the polio and hep B vaccines.

In older kids, it's often given with the Tdap, HPV, and Menactra ® vaccines. Avoid.

Score: -2

Question 4: Are there ways to protect against the disease without getting the vaccine?

Sure. Wash you hands often with soap and water for a good twenty seconds several times a day. Cover your mouth when you sneeze. Disinfect shared surfaces and children's toys. Don't share kitchen items with sick kids. Breastfeed, because you may have antibodies to previous bouts of influenza (another reason for females not to get the influenza vaccine so they can develop actual and lasting immunity to give to their babies via breastfeeding). Keep infants at home during the first few months of life. Select a preschool with fewer students (see Part III). And don't assume that sniffles, stomach distress, or a fever are influenza. They're just as likely to be caused by respiratory syncytial virus, rhinoviruses, or even allergies.

If you do get actual influenza, realize that exercising your immune system is not the worst thing in the world.

Score: -1

OVERALL REWARD-RISK RATING: -4

Public health officials continue to flail and fail when it comes to keeping mercury away from human beings, especially those most senstive to its effects: children and pregnant women. While the sources of exposure are generally well known—eating certain fish, living near point sources of mercury like coal-fired power plants, getting dental amalgams, and receiving thimerosal-containing shots—each is a flashpoint where special interests have set up roadblocks to wise action.

Yet the evidence linking mercury to fetal harm is compelling and cumulative:

- A study found one in six pregnant women had a high-enough mercury load to cause damage to the fetus. Eerily, another study found one in six US children has a neurodevelopmental problem; rates of asthma are in the same range.

- A 2010 publication in *Pediatrics* led by CDC officials reported an elevated risk of autism (nearly double, but not quite statistically significant) from thimerosal-containing shots in pregnant women and infants.

- There's evidence prenatal injections of RhoGAM®, which contained thimerosal, were a contributor to the escalating rates of autism and other neurodevelopmental disorders, like tics, in the 1990s.

- Two studies in Texas pointed to closer proximity to coal-fired plants as doubling the risk of autism in infants.

- A study of air quality in the San Francisco Bay area in 2006 found that children with autism were 50 percent more likely to be born in neighborhoods with high levels of several toxins, particularly mercury.

- Amalgam fillings—mercury mixed with other metals—add to the background load of mercury the mother is carrying. The body naturally tries to detoxify itself, and for a pregnant woman, that means through the fetus. It's well established that mercury levels that have no health impact on the mother can be catastrophic for her offspring. After the Minamata, Japan organic-mercury spill, mothers who showed no effects gave birth to gravely disabled children. For those reasons, it's a good idea not to have dental work done around pregnancy or to have mercury fillings removed then. (It's a good idea not to get mercury fillings, period.)

- Mercury-containing fish, such as tuna and swordfish, are also a risk. There's a whole body of literature on the effects of fish-eating during pregnancy, including from the Faroe and Seychelles Islands. In 2008, the *Medical Journal of Australia* reported on three boys under the age of three who had up to seven times the "safe" mercury level. "The children, who had all been weaned on fish congee, a type of porridge, had eaten fish up to eight times a week and were being treated for developmental delays or neurological problems," according to the *Sydney Morning Herald*. "One, a two-year-old boy being treated for aggressive behavior, ate salmon, barramundi or snapper at least five times a week and had a mercury level three times the safe level. His father had also been diagnosed with mercury poisoning after complaining of rashes, abdominal pain and diarrhea."

Yet the US government still pulls its punches. In 2014, the FDA issued draft wording for advice to pregnant women: "Eat 8 to 12 ounces of a variety of fish each week from choices that are lower in mercury. The nutritional value of fish is important during growth and development before birth, in early infancy for breastfed infants, and in childhood." The FDA listed light, canned tuna as lower in mercury.

Consumer Reports dissented. The magazine—which has no advertising—"disagrees with the recommendations from the FDA and EPA on how much tuna women and children may eat. We don't think pregnant women should eat any."

If you're like most moms and worry about taking care of your baby, you focus on several smart, basic steps—not smoking, eating organic food, shunning alcohol—that are aimed at keeping toxins at bay. Given all these things you do to protect your baby, why would you want a flu shot?

CHAPTER 9

THE ENTERIC VACCINES

- Rotavirus
- Poliovirus
- Hepatitis A

ENTEROVIRUSES ARE A GROUP of more than one hundred viruses that can cause stomach pain, diarrhea, respiratory illness, rash, and, in the case of poliovirus, paralysis and death. They usually replicate in the gastrointestinal (GI) tract—*entero* is from the Greek enteron, or intestine.

While most enterovirus infections are inapparent or cause minor symptoms, the virus can sometimes spread to other organs in the body and trigger severe illness, including aseptic meningitis and encephalitis.

In late 2014, Enterovirus 68 made headlines for causing severe respiratory distress in children, especially those with asthma. There were also scattered reports of paralysis. We suspect enteroviruses, like many other microbes, can be made more virulent by co-factors such as environmental toxins and pesticides, an idea we will discuss in the polio section.

Rotavirus

There's something truly maddening about the rotavirus vaccine: It isn't needed where it's used, and it isn't used where it's needed. The reason is that people with too much power over vaccine recommendations in the United States got it approved here, but the companies they got it approved for have priced the vaccine so high that it's too expensive for consumers in poorer countries. While that may be changing, it's a real window into the way the vaccine schedule in the United States has been hijacked by special interests for whom money is an inevitable part of the reward-risk calculation.

Before we address this unhealthy state of affairs, let's sift through the mass of verbiage around this (and every other vaccine) for the few nuggets that really matter. Rotavirus, a common stomach bug, is simply not a dangerous disease in a place like the United States. The usual scare fest about deaths and hospitalizations masks the truth. Ailments that cause far worse problems get far less attention—there's just no vaccine market for most of them.

Any child's death is tragic; when the numbers are small in relative terms, though, a vaccine needs to be extraordinarily safe so as not to cause more problems than the disease itself. And the time and effort required to prevent a particular disease in a particular population with a particular vaccine needs to be objectively assessed. Rotavirus vaccine flunks those tests big time and lands deep in the red on our Reward-Risk Rating, down there close to Gardasil® as a really, really bad vaccine for American children.

The truth is that in their candid moments, even public health officials don't get too excited about rotavirus. Only West Virginia and North Dakota make it a school requirement. Only a handful of other countries recommend it. Where is the sense of alarm about the lurking menace of rotavirus in the US? Nowhere outside the often-interchangeable offices of drug companies and CDC officials, it seems.

On our blog, Age of Autism, autism parent and Generation Rescue cofounder J. B. Handley wrote about his experience with Oregon health officials in a post titled "Rotavirus: The Vaccine Nobody Wants":

> I found the Department of Health to be extremely helpful in explaining why certain vaccines were not on their required list and in giving me general advice about immunization strategy. When it came to rotavirus, the last vaccine I asked them about, I will just leave you with a quote from their spokesperson: "[A brief chuckle] Well, rotavirus is just some diarrhea for a day or two. It's just not a big deal. That one will never be on our list."

The kicker is that the rotavirus vaccines have turned out to be dangerous and dirty. Dangerous because they can trigger a rare-but-terrible intestinal disorder: intussusception, in which the bowel telescopes in on itself. It is excruciatingly painful, requires hospitalization and surgery, and frequently causes death.

The first vaccine to hit the market, RotaShield®, in 1998, was withdrawn after a year because it clearly caused intussusception that led to deaths—in other words, not before children who didn't need the vaccine died from it. It's the first vaccine ever pulled from the US market.

Merck's RotaTeq® was introduced in 2006, and GlaxoSmithKline came up with Rotarix® a year later. These currently marketed vaccines also appear to cause intussusception, based on reports to VAERS. Cases involving intussusception disappeared when RotaShield® was withdrawn, but then came back in force with RotaTeq®. It would appear the vaccine establishment has gotten its act together since RotaShield® was pulled, finding ways to minimize the risk as a "background rate" that would occur without the vaccine. Nonetheless, it persists.

ROTAVIRUS VACCINES DRIVE INTUSSUSCEPTION EVENTS

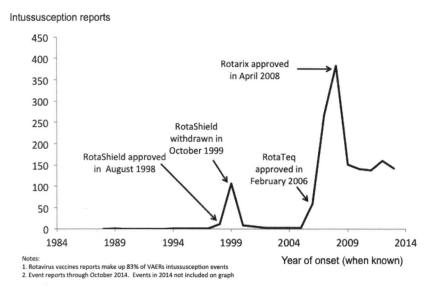

Notes:
1. Rotavirus vaccines reports make up 83% of VAERs intussusception events
2. Event reports through October 2014. Events in 2014 not included on graph

And the vaccine is dirty: so-called adventitious agents—things that shouldn't be there—have now popped up in both RotaTeq® and

Rotarix®. This sounds like a bad joke: they found a pig virus in one of the vaccines, Rotarix®, and decided to suspend its use, but then they found *two* pig viruses in the RotaTeq® vaccine. Well, you can't suspend one and not the other. So the people who advise the CDC on which vaccines every child in America should get decided to keep on giving both.

As we said—it's maddening.

Rotarix®, a liquid, is also known as RV1, because it carries one strain of rotavirus. Made by GlaxoSmithKline, RotaTeq®, a powder that's used to mix an injection, is known as RV5 for targeting five strains of the rotavirus.

Both are recommended at two and four months, with a third shot of RotaTeq® recommended at six months.

Reward Factors

Question 1: How bad is the disease?

Rotavirus is a common cause of childhood diarrhea; it's not that dangerous a disease in a country like the United States. Without vaccination, most kids get it at some point. Rarely, cases can become severe and result in hospitalization or even death. But this illness is the lowest in severity we give to any of the sixteen diseases on our chart.

The CDC Pink Book, a compendium of diseases and vaccines, says that before the vaccine, 95 percent of children had at least one rotavirus infection at some point.

As the Mayo Clinic puts it, "Although rotavirus infections are unpleasant, you can treat most of them at home with extra fluids to prevent dehydration. Occasionally, severe dehydration requires intravenous fluids in the hospital. Dehydration is a serious complication of rotavirus and a major cause of childhood deaths in developing countries."

Score: 0

Question 2: Does getting the vaccine help protect others from getting the same illness?

The vaccine does provide some, modest benefit in protecting others. The virus is easily spread in day care or through interactions with anyone harboring an active infection. But children still get diarrhea, and it's hard to know what percentage of that might be due to rotavirus.

GAVI, the global vaccine alliance, says it is helping introduce the rotavirus vaccine into other countries: "Since 2011, Sudan, Ghana, Rwanda, Moldova, Yemen, Malawi, Armenia, Tanzania, Georgia, Haiti, The Gambia, Burkina Faso, Ethiopia, Zambia and Burundi have introduced rotavirus vaccines into their national immunization programs. Fifteen other countries are expected to introduce rotavirus vaccines in the next two years with Gavi support."

It is in countries like that where almost all the estimated 450,000 deaths from rotavirus occur (the US total is a hundredth of a percent of that). Now seventeen years after the vaccine was introduced (and American children paid the price when it caused intussusception and had to be withdrawn), it may finally be reaching markets that actually might benefit from it.

However, do they want a vaccine known to cause intussusception, contain pig viruses, and target just a few of the many strains of the rotavirus? Would GAVI be wiser and more compassionate to invest in clean water for these developing countries? We think yes.

Score: +3

Question 3: What is the risk of infection?

It's a common bug—the most frequent cause of diarrhea in babies and children around the world, the CDC says. If you don't vaccinate your child, there's a good chance he or she will get it. Like "the flu," stomach bugs can come from many different viruses; just because your child has diarrhea doesn't mean he got the rotavirus.

Score: +4

Question 4: How well does the vaccine work?

In one study, Rotarix® reduced severe rotavirus gastroenteritis by 85 percent. Still, the overall effect is hard to gauge since diarrhea remains a common childhood ailment. The CDC says that the vaccine has resulted in sixty-five thousand fewer children hospitalized, reducing healthcare costs by almost $280 million.

There are dozens of strains of rotavirus, and it's not obvious what percentage of of those strains the vaccines are preventing.

Score: +2

Risk Factors

Question 1: What are the vaccine's side effects?

They're far too serious for the disease the vaccines are trying to prevent. As we noted above, the first vaccine, called RotaShield^R, was pulled within a year after causing intussusception. The two vaccines approved since then also show spikes in the VAERS data for the same problem. While officials try to dismiss that as a background rate, there are scant reports of other vaccines causing the same problem and only a handful of reports after the first vaccine was pulled and before the next one was approved.

Adverse-event reports for the current rotavirus vaccines are the highest for any given to infants, according to Gayle DeLong's analysis of VAERS data. Only Gardasil®, for preteens, and the shingles vaccine, for adults, have higher totals.

RotaTeq®'s adverse event-rate per 100,000 recipients is 54.62, Rotarix's is 58.30—a close correspondence that suggests the risk for both is similar and real. (RotaShield®, the withdrawn vaccine formulation, was twice as bad—106.07.)

By contrast, two vaccines introduced long before the liability shield for drug makers have significantly lower rates. The DTaP vaccine has an adverse-events rate of 30.91 per 100,000 recipients; polio, 22.76. Is it really worth taking more than twice the risk to prevent rotavirus than to prevent polio?

Overall, the average ratio of vaccines the FDA licensed before the 1988 injury-liability act took effect is 19.05, according to DeLong; for vaccines approved since, the average ratio is 40.68.

Score: -5

Question 2: What are the risks of chronic/severe illness and death?

The vaccines can cause an additional one to five cases of intussusception for every 100,000 doses given, according to an analysis in the New England Journal of Medicine in 2014.

The circoviruses in both vaccines are also a cause for concern. One of them causes a wasting disease in pigs similar to AIDS in humans, and the overall health risk of such "adventitious agents" is simply unknowable. Said nurse and vaccine-safety advocate Lyn Redwood, "It is impossible for parents to give free and informed consent to a vaccine containing pig virus DNA when their risks are unknown. To continue to administer these vaccines given the impossibility of informed consent is unethical."

In response to the porcine-circovirus finding, Hong Kong withdrew RotaTeq®, while US public health officials kept both vaccines on the market.

Score: -4

Question 3: What are the consequences of using the vaccine in combination with other vaccines?

Rotavirus is part of the logjam of early vaccines—at two and four months for either formulation, and again at six months for RotaTeq®. For anyone looking to dial back this early onslaught, the rotavirus vaccine would likely be the first to go, along with the hep B vaccine. And remember, states don't require rotavirus for school attendance.

Rotarix is a live-virus vaccine; Rotateq is inactivated. In general, live-virus vaccines seem risky to us in combination with other shots. An infant exposed to a mercury-containing influenza vaccine in utero, followed by two more mercury-containing doses at six months, could be at added risk from doses of the live-rotavirus vaccine.

Score: -2

Question 4: Are there ways to protect against the disease without getting the vaccine?

According to the CDC's Pink Book, "Infants younger than three months of age have relatively low rates of rotavirus infection, probably because of passive maternal antibody, and possibly breastfeeding." This suggests breastfeeding as long as possible can be important.

Score: -2

OVERALL RISK-REWARD SCORE: -4

The Big Picture: Dangers and Dollar Signs in Vaccine Development

For many in the vaccine-safety community, hearing the words "rotavirus vaccine" is enough to summon groans, guffaws, eye rolling, or worse, depending on one's favored method of expressing disdain. And many of those expressions are directed at Paul A. Offit, MD.

Offit is an infectious-disease specialist at the University of Pennsylvania with lots of fancy credentials, including a professorship endowed by Merck, and is a co-developer of RotaTeq®, manufactured by Merck. RotaTeq® was recommended for the childhood schedule by the Advisory Committee on Immunization Practices in 2006.

Offit has acknowledged making $6 million from cashing out one portion of his rights to the vaccine's future profits; we estimate his total income from all sources due to his RotaTeq® patents to be north of $10 million. Yet as a member of the CDC's Advisory Committee on Immunization Practices, he helped establish the recommendation for the rotavirus-vaccine category at the same time he held patents on his rotavirus vaccine-invention.

Offit doesn't consider those facts a problem. "I am a co-holder of a patent for a (rotavirus) vaccine. If this vaccine were to become a routinely recommended vaccine, I would make money off of that," Offit told UPI in 2003. "When I review safety data, am I biased? That answer is really easy: absolutely not."

"Is there an unholy alliance between the people who make recommendations about vaccines and the vaccine manufacturers? The answer is no."

We beg to differ: The answer is really easy—yes. The fact that Offit doesn't see this inherent conflict of interest, and that no one in a position to do so stepped in to prevent it, is evidence that decisions on vaccine approval need to be removed from such obviously self-interested parties. Even a congressional committee criticized Offit for voting on vaccine policies while retaining a financial interest in the outcome.

Offit was appointed to ACIP in 1998 and served until 2003. Shortly before his term began, he'd received four patents on a rotavirus vaccine.

Unlike most other patented products, the market for mandated childhood vaccines is created not by consumer demand, but by the recommendation of ACIP. Certainly a vaccine for polio sixty years ago had plenty of demand, but rotavirus was the subject of no such outcry.

In a single vote, ACIP can create a commercial market for a new vaccine that is worth hundreds of millions of dollars in a matter of months. After ACIP approved the addition of Merck's (and Offit's) RotaTeq® vaccine to the childhood-vaccination schedule, Merck's RotaTeq® revenue rose from zero in the beginning of 2006 to $655 million in fiscal year 2008. When one multiplies a price of close to $200 per three-dose series of RotaTeq® by a mandated market of four million children per year, it's not hard to see the commercial value to Merck of favorable ACIP votes.

Before and during his ACIP term, Offit was involved in rotavirus-vaccine-development activities, the value of which ACIP influenced. Shortly before his term began in October 1998, the US Patent and Trademark Office granted Offit's first two patents. *During his ACIP term*, Offit received two additional patents in 2000 and 2001.

Receiving a patent provides the potential, but not the certainty, of financial reward. In most cases, when an inventor's employer receives a patent, the commercial value of the patent award is highly uncertain. In the case of RotaTeq®, the business uncertainty revolved around three factors: (1) the creation and eventual size of the rotavirus-vaccine market, (2) the market share of competing products such as Wyeth's RotaShield® vaccine (since withdrawn), and (3) the success of Merck's clinical trial for RotaTeq® and subsequent FDA approval.

For the first two of these three factors, Offit's ACIP membership gave him a direct opportunity to favorably influence his personal financial stake in RotaTeq®.

Four months before Offit was appointed to the ACIP in October 1998, the committee had voted to give the rotavirus category "Routine Vaccination" status, in anticipation of an FDA approval of RotaShield®. (Oddly, the ACIP made this vote before the FDA approved Wyeth's RotaShield® vaccine on October 1, 1998.)

Shortly after Offit's term began, there were several additional votes involved in establishing the rotavirus-vaccine market, and Offit voted yes in every case. In May of 1999, the CDC published its revised childhood-vaccination schedule, and the rotavirus vaccine was included. This series of favorable votes clearly enhanced the monetary value of Offit's stake in Merck's rotavirus vaccine, which was five years into clinical trials.

Nevertheless, Merck's RotaTeq® vaccine was several years behind Wyeth's RotaShield®, which stood to be the market leader based on its lead in making its way through clinical trials. But when the widespread administration of RotaShield® to infants started producing a high incidence of intussusception, including reports of fatalities, the ACIP was forced to reverse itself. On October 22, 1999, the ACIP voted to rescind its recommendation of the RotaShield® vaccine.

Offit recused himself from this vote, although he participated in the discussion. In the meeting in which the ACIP discussed RotaShield®, Offit remarked, "I'm not conflicted with Wyeth, but because I consult with Merck on the development of rotavirus vaccine, I would still prefer to abstain because it creates a perception of conflict."

CDC records make it clear that Offit was not silent on RotaShield®. By 2001, he was actively advancing a "unique strain" hypothesis, an argument that RotaShield® was formulated in a way that did increase intussusception risk whereas other formulations (e.g. his own RotaTeq®) would not.

In commercial terms, Offit had a clear stake in the earlier RotaShield® decision. As a competitor to RotaTeq®, RotaShield®'s withdrawal provided a financial opportunity for Offit's partner, Merck. Not only did RotaShield's withdrawal give RotaTeq® an opportunity to gain 100 percent of the rotavirus-vaccine market Offit had voted to create (until April 2008, when GlaxoSmithKline's vaccine was approved, Merck held a monopoly on the rotavirus vaccine-market), but the absence of competition enabled Merck to charge a premium price for its vaccine, significantly more than Wyeth had charged for RotaShield®.

With RotaShield® out of the market and the favorable rotavirus-policy precedent established, when the FDA approved RotaTeq® on February 3, 2006, the path to profitability for Merck was set. And for Offit's employer, the Children's Hospital of Philadelphia (CHOP), which had licensed its patent rights to Merck, the value of its patent portfolio soared. Faced with this newly valuable asset, CHOP chose not to take their profits in the form of a series of smaller royalty checks.

Instead, they opted to sell off their rights to the income stream and receive a lump-sum payment in its place. Royalty Pharma—an intellectual-property investment firm that "provides liquidity to royalty owners and assumes the future risks and rewards of owner-ship"—stepped in to pay CHOP for the rights to its Merck royalties. CHOP, in turn, paid Offit a hefty share of the spoils in return for his role as the vaccine's inventor.

Other news organizations, most notably CBS News, have asked Offit to disclose the financial details of his Merck relationship. Offit protested loudly over the CBS News report and went so far as accusing the network's chief Washington investigative reporter at the time, Sharyl Attkisson, of unethical conduct.

"Did [Attkisson] lie about whether or not we provided materials? Of course," Offit claimed in an interview with the *Orange County Register*. He argued that in responding to a CBS News investigation of his financial ties to Merck, he readily provided full details of the payments that CBS asked for, including: "the sources and amounts of every grant he has received since 1980"; "the details of his rela-tionship, and Children's Hospital of Philadelphia's relationship, with pharmaceutical company Merck"; and "the details of every talk he has given for the past three years."

But for once Offit did not have the last word. The *Register* printed a subsequent correction that began, "Upon further review, it appears that a number of Dr. Offit's statements, as quoted in the *OC Register* article, were unsubstantiated and/or false. . . .

"Documents provided by CBS News indicate Offit did not disclose his financial relationships with Merck, including a $1.5 million Hilleman Chair he sits in that is co-sponsored by Merck. . . . The CBS News documentation indicates Offit also did not disclose his share of past and future royalties for the Merck vaccine he co-invented. To the extent that unsubstantiated and/or false claims appeared in the *OC Register* and have been repeated by other organizations and individuals, the *OC Register* wishes to express this clarification for their reference and for the record."

So far, the two rotavirus vaccines have made their makers $1.3 billion. This is how your child's vaccine cake is baked, parents. Be careful how you slice it.

A final note: Offit has become a leading critic of the theory that vaccines cause autism, another debate in which he has a financial interest. This conflict is ignored by mainstream media outlets that trot him out as the voice of reason against parents who have seen their children become sick and regress after vaccination.

Nice work if you can get it.

Poliovirus

No other disease struck terror in twentieth-century parents like polio— or, to be precise, poliomyelitis. The poliovirus itself appears to have been around for millennia, and only led to outbreaks of paralysis and death beginning in the late nineteenth century.

These episodic outbreaks grew in frequency and size and became a modern scourge when, in 1916, an epidemic caused nine thousand cases with 2,343 deaths in New York City alone. By the early 1950s, several thousand children were infected and many died every year in what became known as "the summer plague" for its predictable arrival and retreat.

Scientists went to work on a vaccine, and in 1955, church bells rang out across the country as Jonas Salk's inactivated vaccine was launched. In 1962, a live-virus version developed by Albert Sabin was introduced—taken in the sugar cubes that many grade school children now past fifty remember well (it seemed a lot better than shots). But that live version was shown to cause polio in around one person per million, and a new, inactivated vaccine was introduced in United States, though the live-virus is still used in other countries.

Polio has now been wiped out in the United States and remains endemic in just three countries—Pakistan, Afghanistan, and Nigeria. But it continues to pop up in places where public health and sanitation break down, most recently in Syria during its civil war.

In our view, the polio vaccine clearly ended the epidemic in the United States and most of the rest of the world. Some in the vaccine-safety community disagree. They believe that polio was already on the decline, that many cases previously diagnosed as polio paralysis are now simply redefined as "flaccid paralysis," and that polio was never an infectious disease at all but was triggered instead by the rise of modern pesticides.

Lost in the heroic narrative of the conquest of the poliovirus is the fact that polio was a dirty vaccine, filtered through primate-kidney tissue; one controversial theory holds that a tainted vaccine-manufacturing process was the cause for the species jump of HIV from chimpanzees to humans. Regardless of whether that's true, it is certainly plausible and indicates the kind of company vaccine ingredients can keep.

Simian Virus 40 definitely made that jump and infected millions of baby boomers with what may be a time bomb—a cancer-causing virus injected into them as children.

Based on our own investigation of polio outbreaks, which we have written about, we propose the rise of polio epidemics may have been due to a combination of pesticide exposure and polio infection. When the virus was circulating in a community and a child was infected with the bug, it would normally either cause a minor infection or pass completely unnoticed.

But if a child ate fruits or vegetables with pesticide residue, the chemicals could open a path for the virus to enter the nervous system and reach the anterior horn cells at the top of the spinal column that control movement—hence, poliomyelitis, a polio infection of the myelin, or gray matter, of the nervous system. Initially, we propose, lead arsenate triggered outbreaks in the 1890s; its successor, DDT—the highly toxic pesticide—led to the big epidemics after World War II.

Poliomyelitis epidemics were unheard of before the 1890s. So the outbreaks of the twentieth century, we believe, were man-made, and the triumph of the vaccine needs to be understood in that light. Nonetheless, it ended a modern plague that is no longer a threat to our children. (We suspect the increased severity and prevalence in 2014 of Enterovirus 68, and particularly the reports of paralysis, may also suggest pesticides or other manmade toxins as a co-factor.)

Now the question becomes, is polio really necessary as a universal childhood vaccine in the United States?

Reward Factors

Question 1: How bad is the disease?

Poliovirus as a stomach bug is benign, but when it resulted in poliomyelitis—in about one in one hundred cases—it was devastating. Although some children recovered completely, many were left with useless arms or legs. Others, whose breathing was paralyzed, suffered for weeks, months, or even years in iron lungs, and most succumbed eventually.

Score: +4

Question 2: Does getting the vaccine help protect others from getting the same illness?

No, not in the United States. Back in the 1950s and 60s, you were protecting your neighbor. But because the disease is no longer circulating, the chances of contracting the illness and then passing it to someone else is virtually zero. The chance of any one person being infected in that way is infinitesimal, and if cases were in fact detected in the US, the vaccine is available.

Score: 0

Question 3: What is the risk of infection?

The last reported case of polio in the United States was in 1979. The risk comes from being unvaccinated and traveling to an area of the world where the virus is still endemic, particularly Africa.

Score: 0

Question 4: How well does the vaccine work?

The killled vaccine appears to be effective. The live-virus vaccine has failed numerous times in areas of the world where the virus still circulates. Some children had to be given the vaccine—which now comes in drops—multiple times before they became immune. This may be because co-factors like the ones we've identified in previous outbreaks are still potentiating the virus in those regions of the world.

Score: +3

Risk Factors

Question 1: What are the vaccine's side effects?

Among the traditional vaccines, polio's side effects are relatively high. The vaccine contains antibiotics, which can trigger allergic reactions. The CDC cites a sore a spot at the injection site as a possibility, but says most people don't have any problems. "However, any medicine could cause a serious side effect, such as a severe allergic reaction or even death." That's extremely rare, the CDC says, but apparently worth mentioning. And it's worth considering in light of the virtually zero possibility of contracting the disease.

Score: -2

Question 2: What are the risks of chronic/severe illness and death?

The oral-polio vaccine—no longer in use in the United States—was in rare cases a cause of paralytic polio itself. According to Gayle

DeLong's analysis, the inactivated vaccine currently in use has the highest rate of adverse events among the pre-NCVIA vaccines, second only to the problematic DTP.

Score: -3

Question 3: What are the consequences of using the vaccine in combination with other vaccines?

At 2, 4, and 6 months, polio vaccine doses are in the logjam of the early-childhood schedule. If, for example, you decided to get the DTaP vaccine during that period because pertussis is a circulating microbe, but were worried about the number of vaccines administered in infancy, the polio vaccine might be eliminated on the premise that it is not a real risk.

Score: -2

Question 4: Are there ways to protect against the disease without getting the vaccine?

Yes, avoid travel to endemic areas of the world. Eat organic food. Sanitation, clean water, pesticide-free food, and other public health measures might do more to contain the virus worldwide than mass-vaccination campaigns.

Score: -1

REWARD-RISK RATING: -1.

Hepatitis A Vaccine

The hepatitis A vaccination shares features with several other vaccines that don't rank high on our Reward-Risk Rating:

- Like rotavirus, catching the disease isn't much of a threat to children. The disease in infants and preschoolers is so mild as to go undetected most of the time.
- Like hep B, it isn't necessary to vaccinate babies to achieve the public health goal of preventing serious hep A disease.
- Like mumps, it's a more serious disease in teens and adults.

Hepatitis A is transmitted via fecal matter, which is why it is both a risk in day care—unwashed hands after a diaper change can spread it all over the place—and among surfers if they come in contact with raw sewage from a municipal wastewater spill on a beach. You can catch it if you travel abroad, if you work with primates, or engage in risky sexual or drug-taking behaviors. You can also catch it at a restaurant from food workers, part of the reason for the ubiquitous "Employees Must Wash Hands Before Returning to Work" signs. Hep A prevention, in fact, is a testament to the power of handwashing and basic hygiene as the single best step towards personal and public disease prevention.

The virus affects the liver and causes inflammation. That's why jaundice is sometimes present. Although it shares its first name with hep B, it is nothing like its far more serious cousin in terms of morbidity and mortality.

That contrast is apparent in states' school-admission policies. While all but three states require hep B vaccinations, the hep A vaccine recommendations resemble Swiss cheese (see chart in Part III): only twenty-one states have it on their school requirements. And in a recent survey of developed countries, only one other country (Monaco) required it.

Most kids under six usually show no symptoms; for the third who do, it looks like a mild flu. This is the reverse of hep B, which is worse in infants, in whom it can become chronic and deadly. From six to twelve, hep A is still mild, although kids may feel sick; past age twelve, it feels like a really bad stomach flu that can go on for weeks.

Rare, severe cases may require rehydration in the hospital for vomiting and diarrhea, accompanied by weight loss and jaundice. Death from hep A is exceedlingly rare, especially among those targeted for vaccination.

Yet like all vaccines—there are two standalone shots for hep A, Havrix by GlaxoSmithKline and Vaqta by Merck—it has the risk of serious reactions. In Gayle DeLong's analysis, hep A does rank fairly low among post-NVCIA vaccines in terms of adverse events per 100,000 recipients—22.08 versus the average 40.68, with a death ratio of 0.037 compared with 0.0826 for all vaccines approved after 1988. But should we really be talking about serious events or death *at all* in a vaccine for an illness that poses virtually no risk to the ones who are getting the injections?

Hep A is a classic post-NCVIA vaccine: not really needed when and where it's given (in infancy, in the US) but capable of doing harm ("unavoidably unsafe") and on a collision course with other vaccines. Parents looking for one to drop could look here; those who want to stick with it might want to wait until a later age.

Reward Factors

Question 1: How bad is the disease?

The CDC says hepatitis A is "a serious liver disease" found in the liver and passed on through the stool of those infected with it and "a person who has hepatitis A can easily pass the disease to others within the same household." The disease can cause flu-like illness, jaundice, and, in children, stomach pains and diarrhea. One in five of those with hepatitis A has to be hospitalized, adults may be out of work for up to a month, and the mortality rate is 3–6 deaths per 1,000 cases, the CDC says.

Score: +1

Question 2: Does getting the vaccine help protect others from getting the same illness?

Yes, infants who are vaccinated cannot pass hep A on via contact with their stool. Vaccinating infants largely benefits older people in whom the disease can be more severe if they haven't caught it in childhood and aren't vaccinated.

Score: +1

Question 3: What is the risk of infection?

The risk of coming down with hepatitis A used to vary a lot by region, with infections occuring far more commonly in the western US. Recently those rates have equalized. Hepatitis A infections often come without symptoms, and reported cases have fallen from 20,000–30,000 annually to below 2,000. Historically, about three quarters of the US population lived through a hepatitis A infection at some point in their lives, but much of the risk occurs later in life. The risk for infants is low.

According to the CDC: "Groups at increased risk for hepatitis A or its complications include international travelers, men who have sex with men, and users of illegal drugs. Outbreaks of hepatitis A have also been reported among persons working with hepatitis A infected primates."

Hep A is the most common illness contracted by Americans traveling abroad and is on the WHO's List of Essential Medicines, and a basic universal vaccination for national health programs. (Do keep in mind that the WHO also states that multiple injections containing the organic mercury preservative, thimerosal, are safe for all children at any age and delivers tens of milliions of such vaccinations to developing countries every year.) As is often true, the case for vaccinating travelers or residents of other countries is completely different from supporting its role on the CDC childhood-immunization schedule.

Score: +1

Question 4: How well does the vaccine work?

It appears to be effective, requiring only two doses a few months apart in infancy—no preschool boosters or adult shots required. Contrast that with the multiple diphtheria, pertussis, and tetanus shots starting in utero and extending for decades.

Score: +4

Risk Factors

Question 1: What are the vaccine's side effects?

The CDC's Vaccine Information Statement says that 1 out of 6 kids (and 1 out of 2 adults—who are more sensitive to the disease itself) will have soreness at the injection site. One out of 25 children (and 1 in 6 adults) will have headache. 1 out of 12 children may lose their appetite.

Severe problems include allergic reactions within a few minutes to hours, which the CDC says are very rare.

Score: -1

Question 2: What are the risks of chronic/severe illness and death?

According to DeLong's analysis, out of 19 million vaccine recipients from 1995 when the vaccine was licensed through 2011, there were 331 reported hospitalizations for vaccine reactions and 20 deaths. That's a small number—but compare it to 501 hospitalizations for the disease in the target population in the year before the FDA licensed the vaccine and only 3 deaths.

DeLong's conclusion, cited in Part 1, is that "a vaccine recipient has a greater probability of reporting a serious adverse event from a vaccine than an unvaccinated person of experiencing a serious side effect from the disease in the year before the FDA licensed the vaccine."

Score: -3

Question 3: What are the consequences of using the vaccine in combination with other vaccines?

The first dose is recommended as early as 12 months. Also recommended at that visit are the MMR combination and chicken pox vaccines, both of which are live-virus shots. The hep A vaccine is recommended between 12 months and 23 months, with 6 months between doses, so if you decide to get it, you might want to move the first dose to the later end of the recommended range.

Score: -2

Question 4: Are there ways to protect against the disease without getting the vaccine?

Yes, this disease is passed along through fecal-oral transmission, so washing your hands is the best defense against infection. If you are exposed, there's no effective treatment except rest and symptom relief.

Score: -1

OVERALL REWARD-RISK RATING: 0

CHAPTER 10

THE EARLY BACTERIAL VACCINES

- Diphtheria equals D
- Tetanus equals T
- Pertussis equals P

3 months of age
ONLY this shot at visit

THE THREE-IN-ONE DTAP VACCINATION is given to protect children against diphtheria, tetanus, and pertussis, a disease better known as whooping cough. In the 1990s, the whole-cell pertussis vaccine in the original DTP shot was replaced with a safer, acellular version—the "a" in DTaP. This was done approximately fifteen years after a US study showed the DTaP vaccine was safer than the DTP shot. Japan immediately altered their vaccine schedule based on the American study, but our government chose to disregard this important safety discovery.

Few vaccines are as widely recommended as DTaP. Every state "mandates" it for public school attendance, and most other countries recommend it, too. The DTP shot, along with the polio and smallpox vaccines, comprised the entire immunization schedule for the majority of the baby boom generation.

We call this trio the early bacterial vaccines—as opposed to the trio of bacterial-meningitis vaccines added later—because they were among the first used in mass-vaccination campaigns. The pertussis vaccine was approved in 1915, the diphtheria vaccine in the late 1920s, and tetanus vaccine a decade later. A combined diphtheria-and-tetanus shot was licensed in 1947, and the combination of those two with pertussis was approved in 1949.

All three of the diseases the DTaP shot is intended to prevent are serious and can be fatal. At the time they were introduced, we would agree, these vaccines made a positive contribution toward reducing the spread of these diseases and saving children's lives.

Diphtheria can lead to the growth of a membrane across the throat that can suffocate its victim, along with causing body-wide complications. Pertussis, or whooping cough, is especially serious in infants; the severe and chronic coughing can lead to brain damage and death. Tetanus leads to a symptom commonly known as "lockjaw," alongside generalized muscle rigidity, and can also kill. By most accounts, the widespread administration of these vaccines reduced the burden of these dangerous diseases.

The question now is whether every child should get every one of these vaccines, several times over, starting in utero and extending through infancy into late adulthood. We believe that for many parents who think about it carefully, the answer may be no, except possibly for the pertussis vaccine. Ironically, given the alphabet soup of D, T, and P combinations, there is no stand-alone shot for pertussis, which would be the most compelling choice of the three when considering the real risk to public health.

The DTaP vaccine is recommended as a five-shot series at 2, 4, 6, 15–18 months, and 4–6 years; the fourth shot can be given as early as 12 months if 6 months have elapsed since the last one. For children who might be sensitive to reactions to the pertussis component, the DT shot is recommended.

There are two versions of DT vaccine, both made by Sanofi; one contains thimerosal, so be sure to get the one that doesn't.

A different formulation of the same vaccines called the Tdap vaccine is recommended for all pregnant women between 27 and 36 weeks, and as a one-time shot at 11–12 years. (A lowercase d, t, or p reflects a reduced dose of those ingredients.)

After that, a Td vaccine (commonly referred to as "a tetanus shot") is recommended every ten years. There's also a standalone tetanus shot, TT, that contains thimerosal, so avoid that one. And there are several combination shots incorporating the DTaP vaccine: Pentacel®, which includes Hib and polio vaccines; Pediarix®, with hep B and polio vaccines; Kinrix®, with DTaP and polio vaccines; and TriHibit®, which adds a Hib vaccine.

There are two DTaP vaccine brands: Daptacel®, by Sanofi Pasteur, which contains a saline (saltwater) solution, 2-phenoxyethanol, aluminum, glutaraldehyde, and formaldehyde; and Infanrix by GlaxoSmithKline, which contains a saline solution, aluminum, polysorbate 80, formaldeyhyde and, in the production process, glutaraldeyhyde.

In both formulations, the diphtheria and tetanus components are grown in cultures. The toxins are removed, and the remainder is purified with formaldehyde. The acellular-pertussis component is grown in a culture, then broken up, and elements are extracted for the vaccine before being filtered and purified. Formaldehyde and glutaraldehyde inactivate the toxins.

The Tdap vaccine is manufactured by Glaxo as Boostrix® (branding the idea of your "tetanus booster"), and by Sanofi as Adacel®. The ingredients are similar to their DTaP vaccine formulations; Boostrix® has less aluminum.

The CDC says "getting diphtheria, tetanus, or pertussis disease is much riskier than getting DTaP vaccine," but acknowledges the shot can cause problems. Mild reactions include fever, redness, swelling, and soreness or tenderness at the injection site in about one in four children, more often after the fourth or fifth dose. Sometimes after those shots, the arm or leg in which the shot was given can swell for up to a week in about one child in thirty.

Mild problems also include fussiness (1 in 3), tiredness or poor appetite (1 in 10), and vomiting (1 in 50), usually within one to three days of the shot.

Moderate, uncommon problems include seizure (jerking or staring) in 1 in 14,000 children, crying nonstop for more than three hours (1 in 1,000), and fever over 105 degrees (1 in 16,000).

Severe, very rare problems incude serious allergic reactions (less than 1 in 1 million), and seizures, coma, or permanent brain damage. The CDC says those reactions "are so rare it is hard to tell if they are caused by the vaccine."

This official list, of course, takes no notice of possible links to autism or other chronic effects like asthma and allergies, which are the subject of thousands of reports to the government's vaccine-safety database.

The DTaP vaccine is widely used in national-vaccine programs around the world. One major difference is that outside the United States, home of the most aggressive vaccination policies, it is often recommended starting at 3 months—a month later than in the US. Evidence suggests this slight delay could make a crucial difference.

Most notably, a study in Manitoba, Canada, in 1995, examined 13,980 children's health records through age seven and found:

- Children whose first dose of the DPT vaccine was delayed by up to one month were "significantly less likely to develop asthma" compared to those who got their first dose by two months old.

- The likelihood of asthma was cut in half if the first dose was not given till the child was older than four months of age.

This is disturbing, given the CDC's own estimate that the lifetime risk of asthma in American children is 13.5 percent and the fact that the rate has been steadily rising. The study's authors note that in Japan, where the first dose is not given until at least three months, the asthma rate is "well below those seen in North America."

Bottom line: Delaying your child's first DTaP shot by one month or more may significantly lower the chance of your child acquiring a lifetime, chronic condition—while providing virtually the same level of protection as following the CDC schedule to the letter.

If that's not an argument for making your own vaccine choices, we don't know what is.

As for autism, the epidemic began around 1988; to that point, the DTP shot was the one routine vaccination that contained the organic-mercury preservative called thimerosal, in a concentration of 25 micrograms. Soon, two more mercury-containing shots—Hib and hep B vaccines—joined the childhood-immunization schedule. That nearly tripled the mercury received in an infant's first year of life, putting it well above the EPA's recommendation, and far beyond any reasonable limit that took into account the precautionary principle. When the problem came to light, an FDA official wrote in an internal e-mail that the agency appeared to have been "asleep at the switch" for years. After an intense debate, the CDC and American Academy of Pediatrics recommended in 1999 that manufacturers phase thimerosal out of all childhood vaccines, and by 2003, it was mostly removed except for multidose flu shots.

While the three-part shot is the primary way to receive the individual D, P, and T vaccines, it's still important to consider the risks and benefits surrounding each of these vaccine doses, and their associated infections, independently.

Diphtheria

A century ago, diphtheria was a terrifying disease—"childhood's deadly scourge," according to a recent history with that title. In New York City alone, "the mortality rate was frightfully high, with children being its most frequent victims. Despite yearly fluctuations, diphtheria was endemic and took a steady toll, claiming more than a thousand deaths per year in the 1890s." Nationwide in 1921, more than 206,000 cases were reported, with 15,000 deaths—a mortality rate five times as high as polio at its peak.

Difficult to treat before the advent of antibiotics (which fight bacteria like diphtheria, tetanus, and pertussis, though not viruses like poliovirus), the disease indeed is frightful. An upper-respiratory infection caught by direct contact or breathing droplets, diphtheria starts as a sore throat. The problem comes when the diphtheria bacterium—*Corynebacterium diphtheriae*—is infected with another microbe that releases a toxin embedded in the diphtheria genes.

This toxin can go on to create a membrane in the throat or sinus cavity that ultimately strangles its victim and often leads to death.

Complications include breathing problems, paralysis, and heart failure, according to the CDC Vaccine Information Statement.

As cases and deaths soared, the medical world raced to find both preventives and treatments. By 1914, a toxin-antitoxin combination—originally used to treat the disease—was adapted to prevent it, with limited success. It combined small doses of the diphtheria toxin itself (a form of vaccination) with protective antibodies (the "antitoxin"). It was a nasty product (the antitoxin was extracted from the blood of infected horses) that required three doses. Parents were prone to skip the followup shots when their child had a reaction to an earlier one.

In 1930, the first diphtheria-toxoid vaccine went into production. By treating the diphtheria toxin with formaldehyde, the toxin was rendered harmless, but the resulting toxoid provoked an immune response that proved sufficient (since more toxoid could be injected than toxin) to protect against the disease without the need for protective antibodies. The new toxoid vaccine required only two doses at first, later reduced to one.

Today, however, a disease that entered the last century as a terrible menace to children is no longer a real threat in this country. Only two cases of diphtheria have been reported in the US since 2000, down from fifty-three between 1980 and 2000. "The most recent reported death in the United States due to respiratory diphtheria was in 2003; a sixty-three-year-old male who had not been vaccinated against diphtheria traveled to Haiti," writes Kristine M. Bisgard, a Commander in the US Public Health Service.

Diphtheria is now much like yellow fever, for which a vaccine also exists but is not on the childhood schedule, and other once-prevalent illnesses—not eradicated, but no threat in the United States.

While the medical establishment likes to credit the diphtheria vaccine for eradication of the disease, the picture is a bit more complicated than that. As is often the case with modern diseases, diphtheria and its associated death toll was on the decline due to better hygiene and sanitation by the time the toxoid vaccine arrived.

DIPHTHERIA MORTALITY RATE: 1900-98

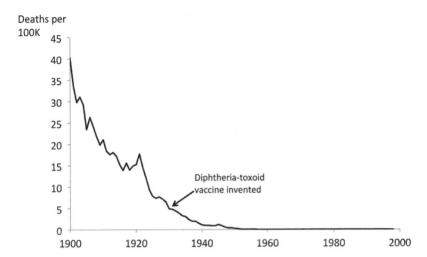

Deaths per 100K

Diphtheria-toxoid vaccine invented

The rise of large cities and the lack of modern sewage control in the late nineteenth century spread deadly scourges; the rise of public health measures like clean water and sewers and the decline of horses and their droppings on city street helped stem them.

"There is no doubt that exposure to sewage emanation is a fruitful source of diphtheria," wrote one observer in 1894. "The statistics of the association between the two are very positive." According to a more recent analysis by Hillary Butler, "There are many historical instances of sewage being relevant to the spread of disease, but even today very few textbooks mention this."

And while cleaning up sewage is a pretty straightforward public health improvement, the introduction of mass vaccination has had unintended consequences rivaling the diseases being attacked. Among the shots on today's crowded CDC vaccine schedule, diphtheria stands out as unnecessary—it prevents a disease that doesn't exist in modern America, and even if it did reappear, a disease treatable by modern medicine.

Question 1: How bad is the disease?

Diphtheria is a serious infection, especially for children, and dangerous in an unusual way. Although it starts with standard symptoms like sore throat, fever, and poor appetite, a toxin secreted by the bacteria creates waste products that slowly build up to form what's called a pseudomembrane. This covers nasal tissues and the larynx and pharynx, obstructing breathing. The bacteria can also damage the heart, inflame the nerves, and cause ear problems.

Overall, the death rate is about 20 percent for children under the age of five and in older people, 5 to 10 percent for those in between.

Score: +4

Question 2: Does getting the vaccine help protect others from getting the same illness?

Back in the 1920s, when diphtheria was endemic in American cities, there was a protective effect both for children who got the vaccine and those they came in contact with. Now, since diphtheria doesn't circulate, you're not doing much to protect your neighbors or fellow-day care students by getting vaccinated for diphtheria. You might be protecting people if you're traveling abroad. That's only a minor argument for vaccination today.

Score: +1

Question 3: What is the risk of infection?

Negligible inside the United States. In the twenty-first century, diphtheria may still be endemic in Haiti (where the last person to die of diphtheria in the United States contracted it; he was unvaccinated) and in Northern Plains Native American reservations, although that is uncertain.

Score: +1

Question 4: How well does the vaccine work?

There are few reports of diphtheria-vaccine failure and little real-world evidence on its efficacy. Perhaps that's evidence that the vaccine has worked well; perhaps it's evidence that fewer horses and cleaner streets have eliminated the conditions that made diphtheria pervasive.

Skeptics of the effectiveness of vaccine programs often point to the decline of diphtheria with the arrival of modern hygiene as a case in point.

Score: +3

Risk Factors

Question 1: What are the vaccine's side effects?

As part of a combination shot, the diphtheria component is inseparable from the pertussis and tetanus vaccines. The pertussis vaccine has gotten most of the attention for its side effects, and that part of the vaccine was changed several years ago to an acellular formulation.

Score: -3

Question 2: What are the risks of chronic/severe illness and death?

The combined DTaP vaccine is linked to encephalitis—brain swelling that causes a characteristic arched back and high-pitched scream. This is often dismissed by pediatricians as "screaming baby syndrome," as if that somehow makes it less concerning.

The newer version, however, has resulted in far fewer reports to the VAERS system—a death rate of 0.0096 per 100,000, as opposed to 1.5648 for the DTP shot, whose severe side effects were largely responsible for the creation of the Vaccine Injury Compensation Act. That's still higher than the average of vaccines licensed after 1988, at 0.0826.

The Tdap vaccine, which contains less diphtheria and pertussis, is in the average range for reported deaths, and the DT shot, with no pertussis, is lower still. This suggests that the diphtheria vaccine by itself might not be a higher-risk vaccine, but in the absence of a great need and the lack of any monovalent vaccine, it's unlikely anyone would ever bother to find out.

Score: -4

Question 3: What are the consequences of using the vaccine in combination with other vaccines?

In addition to being part of a combination shot, the vaccine is given with a number of others, crowded into the first few months of the immunization schedule at 2, 4, 6, and 15–18 months. The safest course would have been a separate pertussis vaccine, since pertussis actually circulates in the United States and is dangerous for a baby to contract. Instead, the DT vaccine is offered to give a non-pertussis option!

Score: -3

Question 4: Are there ways to protect against the disease without getting the vaccine?

Breastfeeding helps protect against infection. If you're worried about diphtheria, stay in the United States. Don't take your child somewhere diphtheria remains endemic. The fact is that anyone going about their business in the US is about as protected from diphtheria as it's possible to be.

Score: 0

OVERALL REWARD-RISK RATING: -1.

The Big Picture: Blindly Fighting Diseases From the Nineteenth Century

Too many vaccines the CDC recommends are no longer essential components of a sensible mass-vaccination policy. Diphtheria is a case in point. The conditions that led to its spread—an endemic bacteria, primitive public health policies, and unsanitary big cities—no longer exist.

The tetanus shot, also part of the DTaP vaccine, makes little sense as a required shot. The common justification for the tetanus vaccine is the so-called "rusty-nail" risk. In actuality, when tetanus was a large problem, it was because horse manure was a major issue for most urban areas and provided a reservoir for tetanus. As general hygiene has improved, the risk of tetanus has gone nearly to zero.

Even the polio vaccine—despite its iconic status and the way it is used to scare people about "a return to iron lungs"—is no longer a necessary protective treatment in twenty-first century America. Polio, which became epidemic in the 1890s but was largely a twentieth-century scourge, is only a threat if you are going to one of the very few, and largely inaccessible, areas of the world where the poliovirus still circulates.

As such diseases have faded, medicine has also added more weapons to its arsenal. Diphtheria can be a dangerous disease, but it can also be mild, and there is antibiotic treatment, so the decision to forego vaccination doesn't leave you helpless in the unlikely event that your child comes down with diphtheria. Antibodies to diphtheria (also known as antitoxins) can be provided, as well as antibiotics.

Antibiotics are widely helpful for many diseases targeted by vaccines. They didn't exist when the mass-vaccination attack on diphtheria began in the 1930s.

Pertussis

The pertussis (whooping cough) vaccine ranks highest on our Reward-Risk Rating. That's because it's a serious disease your child could actually catch today in the United States.

Unlike diphtheria—all but extinct here—pertussis actively circulates in the US. And unlike tetanus, it's a risk for an infected person's close contacts, including infants, in whom it is especially dangerous.

Recent outbreaks in California and elsewhere have made headlines and been fodder for those who say it points to the dangers of vaccine refusal. The flaw in that case is that most of the time, the people who get pertussis are already vaccinated. In one recent study,

81 percent of Californians who came down with pertussis were fully vaccinated and another 11 percent partially vaccinated.

This state of affairs came about after the whole-cell version of the vaccine—which caused severe reactions that led to permanent disability and death—was replaced by a newer, acellular version. This version is clearly not as effective, although it is considerably safer.

There is also the matter of the genetic "drift" of the bacteria itself, perhaps mutating in response to the vaccine in a way that creates a new disease, atypical pertussis. Less virulent forms of the disease producing persistent-but-milder coughing may go unreported, suggesting that even reported rates of pertussis might underestimate the problem. (A study in vaccinated baboons showed that the vaccinated can harbor the pertussis bacteria in their throats for quite some time and spread it to others, even if asymptomatic.)

Nonetheless, whooping cough is a dangerous disease for a child to get, and as long as the bacteria is a real threat, vaccinating against it is a reasonable option. It's unfortunate that the vaccine isn't better and that no single pertussis vaccine exists—no P standing alone amid the forest of D's and T's, because it is the one with, by far, the strongest argument for giving to your infant.

Reward Factors

Question 1: How bad is the disease?

Pertussis in adults can be painful, annoying, and hard to treat. With healthy people, pertussis leads to a few weeks of a nasty cough but is generally not fatal. In fact, the disease is probably circulating widely and its signs often unrecognized—a persistent cough that goes untested or unreported, or which results in no symptoms at all.

In children under six months of age, pertussis is particularly dangerous, and in the early-twentieth century was a major contributor to childhood mortality. Paroxysmal coughing spells can go on nonstop, breaking bones, disrupting breathing, and causing brain damage.

The CDC reported 18,700 cases of pertussis in 2011—that's a lot—with 2,200 in children less than one year old. There are about fifteen deaths a year, most, presumably, in infants—a modest risk of death, less than 1 percent in infants who contract whooping cough.

Score: +4

Question 2: Does getting the vaccine help protect others from getting the same illness?

The obvious inadequacy of the product suggests that getting the vaccine is not doing as much as it claims for your child or anyone else. Further, the vaccine's effectiveness clearly wanes over time. Still, the bacterium is circulating, and getting vaccinated can help protect infants.

That's the reason they're giving the Tdap vaccine to mothers in pregnancy, to create a cocoon of protection around the infant. But that's a vicious circle—when people used to get pertusssis, the mother's antibodies to the actual illness were protective for her infant.

Now, with mass vaccination, mothers have had their immunity to the disease wane by the time they become pregnant.

Score: +5

Question 3: What is the risk of infection?

Low but increasing. In 2010, California experienced the largest whooping-cough outbreak since 1947, with ten deaths. That was just the start—in June 2014, the state health department declared the disease endemic, citing 3,458 cases from January through June 10, a sharp rise from the year before. Across the country in September, a Maryland school district warned parents that 16 cases had been identified since the school year began.

Score: +2

Question 4: How well does the vaccine work?

Failure rates are high, which helps explains five shots for kids, one for pregnant women, and further boosters in adolescence and throughout life. There is some protection, but not as much as you'd think. One unpublished analysis found, in 2014, that the rate of pertussis seemed higher in populations that were the most heavily vaccinated.

Score: +2

Risk Factors

Question 1: What are the vaccine's side effects?

This shot has a long history of serious side effects, notably encephalitis (brain swelling), which can lead to encephalopathy (brain disease, damage, or malfunction). The new, acellular vaccine appears to have reduced this, but it still happens.

Score: -3

Question 2: What are the risks of chronic/severe illness and death?

Giving the first shot at two months appears to carry a real risk of asthma development and, presumably, other chronic conditions. Waiting even a month or two for the first shot shows a significant improvement in the risk.

The DTaP vaccine, although safer than its predecessor, is still among the riskiest vaccines, with a reduction of adverse event rates of only 21 percent, hardly a safety revolution.

It's worth remembering that the DTP vaccine led to the creation of the Vaccine Injury Compensation Program. Note well: It was parental pressure, not proactive efforts by the vaccine industry, that got the vaccine formulation changed to the acellular version. (And remember, the US government sat on safety information for nearly fifteen years before acting on it.)

Score: -4

Question 3: What are the consequences of using the vaccine in combination with other vaccines?

You don't get a pertussis shot without a combination of tetanus and/ or diphtheria. It's almost always given with other early vaccines on the childhood schedule; if you decide to get it, you could consider making it the only injection at that well-baby visit, or perhaps allow just one more, in the other arm or thigh, to link any local-vaccine reaction to a particular shot. The habit of giving multiple needle jabs at once, ostensibly to keep a child from repeated discomfort, is not really in their best interest.

Score: -3

Question 4: Are there ways to protect against the disease without getting the vaccine?

For infants, extended breastfeeding can be protective; if the mother has had pertussis, she can pass along immunity. Ironically, the current wave of pertussis outbreaks might be reestablishing a form of natural immunity in young women who contract wild-type pertussis and, along with that, protective antibodies for a future infant.

Score: 0

OVERALL REWARD-RISK RATING: 3.

The Big Picture: Vaccine Injury Is All Too Real

The origins of the NCVIA go back to the vaccine with the most troubled early safety record, the DwPT (known as the DPT or DTP) vaccine; the w stands for whole-cell. The telltale signs of DwPT vaccine injuries were unmistakable. They also motivated the shift to DTaP vaccines.

The medical literature is full of examples of this, and an early consensus emerged that families deserved to be compensated. Lawsuits over DwPT vaccines led to threats on the part of some vaccine manufacturers to withdraw from the market.

More recently, some industry advocates, and journalists like Brian Deer, have spearheaded a campaign to deny instances of vaccine injury. It's reminiscent of the way drug companies fought off suits for damage from Vioxx and, before that, tobacco—while there was a scientific consensus that the product could cause the injury being alleged, the manufacturers fought tooth and nail to raise doubt it caused the individual plaintiff's injury or death.

The most prominent vaccine-injury denier in the United States, Paul Offit, now denies the previous pertussis vaccine was even a problem. "The modern American anti-vaccine movement was born on April 19, 1982, when WRC-TV, a local NBC affiliate in Washington, D.C., aired a one-hour documentary titled 'Vaccine Roulette.'" Offit portrayed this—rather than the stories of convincing vaccine injury it told—as the root of the DPT vaccine concern that led to a perfectly good vaccine being replaced by one not nearly so good. "It was wrong," Offit said in a 2011 interview. "The whooping cough vaccine didn't cause permanent brain damage, but it had tremendous fallout. It really gave birth to the notion in this country that vaccines might be doing more harm than good."

This kind of vaccine-injury denial kept the switch to the new, safer vaccine from being made for several years, even as Japan and other countries moved to the safer, acellular version. It was a clear case where even at the risk of more pertussis cases, it was worth the reduction in harm from the vaccine itself.

The lesson for those considering any childhood shot is inescapable: vaccines can be dangerous, and resistance to fixing a problem can be unreasonable, especially when a fix is available. Keep that in mind if your doctor tells you vaccine injury almost never, ever, ever happens. It happens all the time.

Tetanus

Tetanus is terrible. First it clenches your teeth in a spasm, the characteristic "lockjaw" that gives the disease its descriptive nickname. The spasm never unlocks, creating the perverse appearance of a grin across the face, even in death, known as *risus sardonicus.*

As other muscles painfully contract, the body arches backward, bones can break, and it becomes impossible to swallow and, finally, from the relentless pressure on the chest, to breathe. With the best of care, 30 to 50 percent of patients with clinical signs of tetanus suffocate and die.

Most horrible is what UNICEF calls the "quick and painful death" of newborns from tetanus as the result of unhygienic birthing practices that allow the bacterium to infect the umbilical cord, which in some parts of the world continue to this day. About 74,000 infants still die every year, mostly in Africa and Southeast Asia.

Tetanus is caused by the bacterium *Clostridium tetani,* which is present in soil, especially cultivated farmland treated with fertilizer; in the guts of animals like cows and pigs; and on dirty objects like the pro-verbial "rusty nail." Puncture wounds are especially dangerous, because they fully enclose the bacterium, which can't survive in air or sunlight.

Once the microbe gets inside, unless treated quickly it produces the most toxic poison known to man, a substance aptly named *tetanospasmin* that blocks the nerve signals that tell muscles to relax.

Tetantus is terrible, but it is also rare in the United States. There are around 50 cases a year, about 1 a year in children under 5, and most of the others in people over 50.

Like diphtheria, tetanus deaths waned as human exposure to its sources diminished and antibiotics and other remedies increased the chances of survival from an infected wound. The disease has all but faded away in developed countries, and the vaccine doesn't offer any "herd immunity" at all—it only protects the person who gets it. Yet more shots than ever containing the tetanus vaccine are on the im-munization schedule.

Tetanus vaccines, in fact, have become a bit of a bait and switch proposition. Many of us accept a longstanding tradition of periodic tetanus boosters, embedded in many hospital-admission protocols and doctor's office routines. The threat of tetanus affecting a wound legitimizes compliance by patients who might otherwise be skeptical of the need for a shot.

The traditional booster vaccines either came in TD or Dt forms. Increasingly, the Tdap vaccine, cunningly branded by GlaxoSmith-Kline as Boostrix® (2013 revenue: $405 million), has become a way for doctors to sneak an additional pertussis vaccine into the schedule.

The Tdap version is now recommended for all pregnant women; the DTaP shot at 2, 4, 6, 18 months, and 4-6 years; the Tdap vaccine again at 11–12 years old, and a Td shot every ten years.

One version of the DT vaccine, and the only version of the standalone tetanus vaccine (TT) contain the ethylmercury preservative thimerosal, which we recommend avoiding at any cost.

Reward Factors

Question 1: How bad is the disease?

"The disease usually presents with a descending pattern," according to the CDC's Pink Book. "The first sign is trismus or lockjaw, followed by stiffness of the neck, difficulty in swallowing, and rigidity of abdominal muscles. Other symptoms include elevated temperature, sweating, elevated blood pressure, and episodic rapid heart rate. Spasms may occur frequently and last for several minutes. Spasms continue for 3–4 weeks. Complete recovery may take months." If it happens.

Score: +5

Question 2: Does getting the vaccine help protect others from getting the same illness?

No. Unlike diphtheria and pertussis, tetanus is caused by infection of an open break in the skin. Getting the shot doesn't protect anyone else—this is the one vaccine on the childhood schedule that has no public health or "herd immunity" value, even in theory. It's infectious but not contagious.

Score: 0

Question 3: What is the risk of infection?

Everyone talks about the rusty-nail risk, but the real problem throughout history has been from animals and particularly horse manure, which used to be a feature of every urban thoroughfare. These risks are sharply reduced in our post-agrarian society where horseless carriages (aka cars) now rule the streets. The CDC notes that the bacterial spores are "widely distributed" in soil that has been treated with manure, as well as in "the intestines and feces of horses, sheep, cattle, dogs, cats, rats, guinea pigs, and chickens."

So someone who works around horses or on a farm or in construction might want to consider it. But the fact is there are a handful of deaths now in the United States from tetanus—from four to six cases a year, a vanishingly small death rate. There were only thirty-six widely distributed cases all told in 2011— one case in New England, one case in the Mid-Atlantic, four cases in Michigan, and three cases in California.

Score: +1

Question 4: How well does the vaccine work?

That's hard to know since actual cases are so few and were falling well before the introduction of the vaccine.

"Several factors have contributed to the decline in tetanus morbidity and mortality, including the widespread use of tetanus toxoid-containing vaccines since the late 1940s," the CDC says. But it acknowledges "other factors include improved wound care management and the use of tetanus immune globulin (TIG) for post-exposure prophylaxis in wound treatment and for the treatment of tetanus. In addition, increased rural-to-urban migration with consequent decreased exposure to tetanus spores may also have contributed to the decline in tetanus mortality noted during the first half of the 20th century."

Among 1,018 cases of tetanus from 1972 to 1979, the CDC says "only" 163 of those, or 16 percent, had three or more vaccine doses. But that—and the need for frequent boosters throughout life— suggests the vaccine is not entirely effective.

Score: +3

Risk Factors

Question 1: What are the vaccine's side effects?

As with all combination vaccines, it's hard to tell in isolation. But given that the risk of the disease is so low, the risk of side effects from the vaccine are actually comparable to getting the disease and dying from it.

Filmmaker Eric Gladen (*Trace Amounts*) said a mercury-containing tetanus shot at age twenty-nine, after he cut himself doing work outside, led to serious long-term health problems. "I hadn't had a tetanus shot in eleven years or so, so I went and got a routine shot," Gladen told KOMO News in Seattle. "Within a few days, some symptoms developed. And then slowly over time, over about three to six months, major neurological symptoms kicked in."

What did Gladen take from the experience? "If I had kids, I would get them vaccinated. But I would do it differently than the current vaccine schedule. I certainly wouldn't give them a vaccine with thimerosal in it. And I wouldn't give them more than one a day."

Score: -3

Question 2: What are the risks of chronic/severe illness and death?

The standalone tetanus shot (TT) contains thimerosal, as does one version of the DT. We advise never getting a thimerosal-containing vaccine. In case of a wound or burn where tetanus is a concern, the CDC says the Td vaccine (trace amounts of thimerosal) can be given.

Score: -4

Question 3: What are the consequences of using the vaccine in combination with other vaccines?

There is an increasing trend toward slipping other components into a "tetanus booster" to pursue other agendas (like failing pertussis vaccines), while pitching the rusty-nail rationale.

Score: -3

Question 4: Are there ways to protect against the disease without getting the vaccine?

Wear strong-soled shoes. Avoid animal waste. Make sure any wound is treated with soap and water and/or hydrogen peroxide and a deep or dirty wound gets prompt medical attention.

Score: -2

OVERALL REWARD-RISK RATING: -3

The Big Picture: Clean Underwear and the Folly of Eradication

The smallpox vaccine is the most successful vaccine in history, its inventor an Englishman named Edward Jenner. That early success stands in stark contrast to the new, high-tech vaccines like Recombivax B® and Gardasil®.

The technology underlying Jenner's smallpox vaccine was primitive. The germ theory of infectious disease was not well understood at the time Jenner began experimenting with his vaccine in 1793. Jenner himself, although universally praised today as a great innovator, was something less than a heroic figure. The second child he vaccinated, a five-year-old named John Baker, died shortly after vaccination. Jenner was a controversial figure in his day, criticized as a "lazy, unmethodical, loose-minded shuffler" who wrote a fraudulent paper on cuckoo birds.

Most importantly, it appears Jenner almost certainly misinterpreted the biological mechanism for his invention and probably misnamed its source, thinking it was cowpox, when it was actually another virus now known as vaccinia. Indeed, the true source of the virus that formed the basis for the modern smallpox vaccine remains a scientific puzzle and an enduring mystery. As much as public health spokespeople love to hold up vaccination as a heroic technological achievement, Jenner's work performs poorly as a triumphant tale of science-based invention.

Jenner's blundering aside, however, by most accounts the smallpox vaccine that resulted from his work became a spectacular success. The death rate from vaccination was much lower than the technique that preceded it, "variolation," directly infecting the patient with variola, the smallpox virus. Most consumers feared the deadly infection and willingly absorbed the risk of vaccination, and the vaccine's widespread adoption was limited more by availability of the product than acceptance of the technology. Consumers embraced the smallpox vaccine with little need for government intervention.

By 1971, the vaccine was removed from the childhood-vaccine schedule in the United States, and the World Health Organization declared the world free of the smallpox virus in October 1979.

However crude the technology for the smallpox vaccine was, its success may never be replicated. The unusual nature of the virus made smallpox an easy target. There was no known disease reservoir—a place outside the human body where a bacteria can grow and multiply—so herd immunity could inexorably lead to eradication. The vaccine that provided immunity wasn't even based on the virus itself, merely a cousin. And the broad immunity derived from this single vaccine strain made it the only virus ever eradicated with vaccination. Bill Gates is working hard to earn a place in history by eradicating polio, but it's not looking good.

Smallpox and polio have something in common; the only reservoir for the disease is humans. The list of diseases that work that way is quite small.

For diseases that are carried by bacteria as opposed to viruses, the importance of public and personal hygiene is too frequently overlooked relative to vaccination. In fact, leading advocates of vaccination today like the Johns Hopkins Bloomberg School of Public Health started out as Johns Hopkins School of Hygiene and Public Health in 1916. Put differently, the benefits of clean underwear and clean streets have had a far greater impact on reducing the burden of infectious disease than vaccines.

With respect to the DTP trio of diseases, it's clear that with improvements in general hygiene over the last century, the risk of diseases like tetanus and diphtheria has gone nearly to zero.

Tetanus is everywhere because it inhabits the intestines of horses and other domesticated animals, but the risk has gone down in large part because exposure to horse manure is greatly reduced. You don't hear many calls to eradicate the bacterium *Clostridium tetani.* Instead, the tetanus vaccine survives as an anachronism, an echo of an obsolete urban economy not much more relevant than a Boston subway stop named "Haymarket" or pubs named "The Carriage House."

Few viruses have only humans as their disease reservoir. Rabies circulates mostly in animals, so no one talks about our responsibilty to protect the herd from rabies. Influenza moves around from birds to pigs to horses to humans and back, so it will be an issue forever; we either make peace with that or keep chasing our tails every year with reminders not to forget our annual flu shot for little real benefit and considerable risk.

It's no accident that the vaccines we have rated the highest in terms of Reward-Risk—pertussis, rubella, and measles—tend also to have the most compelling herd benefit.

CHAPTER 11

THE BACTERIAL MENINGITIS VACCINES

- Haemophilis Influenza B (Hib)
- Pneumococcal
- Meningococcal

LIKE THE DTAP VACCINE, THESE THREE KILLED-virus vaccines protect against bacterial disease, most prominently meningitis. Unlike the DTaP shot, they are administered in separate doses.

The meninges are the membranes that surround and protect the central nervous system. If they become inflamed, either in the brain or spinal cord, a condition called meningitis, the consequences can be catastrophic and deadly.

Hib disease usually affects children younger than five, which is why the vaccine is routinely recommended for day care or preschool, but not for elementary school admission. The vaccine is given at two, four, six, and fifteen months.

Pneumococcal disease generally affects infants under the age of two, and the vaccine is also commonly required in day care settings but not kindergarten and beyond. In addition to causing meningitis in rare cases, it is responsible for the majority of bacterial ear infections in children (most ear infections are caused by viruses). Like the Hib vaccine, it is given at two, four, six, and fifteen months.

Meningococcal disease, which is very rare but can be devastating—leading to death—is most likely in settings such as college and boarding schools where adolescents are in confined quarters. For that reason the vaccine is recommended at eleven or twelve years, with a second dose at age sixteen. Many colleges require it for incoming freshmen, and boarding schools may do so, too.

While they target different bacteria whose only connection is their ability to cause illness, in particular meningitis, these three vaccines share something unique—the way they are made. All three are "conjugate" vaccines. Think of the vaccine as a missing person's coat that a bloodhound is given to sniff before being set loose to find them. In the case of the meningitis vaccines, the telltale piece that primes the immune system to detect the real thing comes from the coating or capsule around the vaccine, which is made of molecules of various sugars—polysaccharides. Historically, vaccines made solely from polysaccharides haven't worked very well—the protection wore off too quickly—so they weren't recommended very often. The only benefit might be for a short trip to an area with high risk of infection.

Enter the new technology. With conjugate vaccines, those target pieces of polysaccharide are obtained from the bacteria themselves and then joined—conjugated—with substances that increase their ability to trigger an immune response. In the case of the pneumococcal vaccine, diphtheria toxoid is added in with the sugars to create the vaccine. For the Hib vaccine, it's tetanus toxoid, and for meningococcus, it's also dipththeria.

This new technology, first introduced with the Hib vaccine in 1988, is reminiscent of the high-tech approaches we describe with hepatitis B (recombinant DNA) and Gardasil® (virus-like particles). While these may smooth the manufacturing process and allow new kinds of vaccinations to enter the market, there's also the possibility that this technique has consequences that have not yet been recognized.

Bacterial meningitis is a bad disease but very rare. It causes death and serious disability in a significant proportion of cases, often 10 percent or more.

These bacteria can also cause other diseases. Hib can cause epiglottitis, pneumonia, arthritis, middle-ear infections, and osteomyelitis. Invasive-pneumococcal disease also leads to pneumonia and some kinds of ear infections (aka acute *otitis media*). Meningococcal disease can also lead to *otitis media*. The reason antibiotics are often given for ear infections, despite the fact that *otitis media* is almost always viral in origin, is that some of the most severe infections can be caused by these bacteria, and pediatricians are practicing defensive medicine. (A 2013 report in *Pediatrics* found that "most upper respiratory tract infections are caused by viruses and require no antibiotics," despite the fact that more than one in five visits to pediatricians result in antibiotic prescriptions—50 million a year!)

These bacteria are pervasive, and the reason they become virulent remains a mystery. There may be some co-factor created by modern medicine or the environment that is potentiating them in certain children.

Another factor to weigh: The risk of getting some types of bacterial meningitis is a bit higher than, but on the order of, a lightning strike. The risk of getting struck by lightning in a given year is one in five hundred thousand. The attack rate of meningococcal meningitis, for example, is 1–3 in 100,000 in the target population for the vaccine, eighteen to twenty-three-year-olds (Hib meningitis rates, by contrast, have been much higher, over 100 per 100,000 in the first year of life). If all meningococcal meningitis came from a single bacterium, then maybe a vaccine strategy would be stronger.

The problems is, there are at least dozens of different bacteria involved, and each individual vaccine only protects against a narrow range. So each vaccination choice balances the risk of an adverse event with an exceedingly rare chance of meaningful protection.

Hib

The Hib vaccine was among the earliest additions following enactment of the vaccine-injury act, and among the least controversial. Hib is a pervasive bacterium that colonizes the nasal passage and is present in a lot of healthy carriers. Somehow, it can get into the bloodstream, though no one knows how, and from there to the meninges. If that happens, one in seven kids have long-lasting issues.

Before the vaccine, the vast majority of kids got immunity to Hib without getting meningitis. This makes the disease a little bit like varicella (chickenpox), mostly benign but with very rare complications.

One reason Hib has received less notoriety than other vaccines is that many different forms of the Hib vaccine hit the market beginning in the late 1980s. Vaccine-adverse events also occur more rarely than other newcomers to the vaccine schedule, but are higher than the traditional vaccines, according to Gayle DeLong's analysis. But despite its relatively benign reputation, some controversial risks may be significant, including an increased diabetes risk and peanut allergy.

Relative to the other meningitis vaccines, the Hib vaccine does have the advantage of targeting just one microbe. Its chances of hitting the most beneficial target are therefore much better than the scattershot approach of the other two vaccines.

Reward Factors

Question 1: How bad is the disease?

Generally mild unless the microbe escapes into the bloodstream. In that case it can cause lasting damage or death. Virginia pediatrician Elizabeth Mumper, who is a supporter of the vaccine, vividly recalls seeing previously healthy infants before the vaccine became available whose spinal fluid was filled with pus.

Score: +5

Question 2: Does getting the vaccine help protect others from getting the same illness?

The microbe appears pervasive in the environment. It mainly protects the person receiving it. The CDC has claimed a sharp reduction in Hib disease, but this may have more to do with direct effects of the vaccine rather than herd immunity.

Score: +1

Question 3: What is the risk of infection?

The infection is already present in the upper-respiratory tract of every human being—the microbiome. It's what allows access to the bloodstream that is mysterious and, fortunately, rare.

Score: +1

Question 4: How well does the vaccine work?

Since it targets just one microbe, it appears to work well enough. The danger from the infection is greatly reduced by the time a child is ready for kindergarten.

Score: +3

Risk Factors

Question 1: What are the vaccine's side effects?

Overall, the side-effect profile is relatively mild—brief fainting spells after injection and, rarely, severe shoulder pain. Severe allergic reactions are less than one in a million, the CDC says.

Score: -1

Question 2: What are the risks of chronic/severe illness and death?

Juvenile diabetes appears to be one. One analysis found that two separate groups of Finnish children with Hib vaccine exposures had higher incidence of diabetes than a group not exposed to the Hib vaccine. Also consistent with their hypothesis, the group receiving 4 doses of the vaccine (at 3, 4, 6, and 18 months) had higher incidences of diabetes than the group receiving only one dose at 24 months. The relative risk for the 4-dose group was 1.26 at 7 years of age and 1.17 at 10 years of age. The increase in incidence was 54–58 per 100,000 children. These were statistically significant results.

Heather Fraser, author of *The Peanut Allergy Epidemic*, believes the vaccine is implicated in the sudden rise of peanut allergy, now affecting 5.6 million people in the United States but unheard of a generation ago.

"The Hib, within an intense schedule that includes five-vaccines-at-once, has been the last straw in my opinion, tipping scores of children into peanut allergy," she writes.

"Medical literature has illustrated that the only means by which mass allergy has ever been created was by injection. With the pairing of the hypodermic needles and vaccines at the close of the 19th century, allergy and anaphylaxis made their explosive entry into the western world.

"Serum sickness from this new procedure was the first mass-allergic phenomenon in history. Epidemic allergy to penicillin reminiscent of the 'days of serum sickness' emerged with its mass application following WWII."

Score: -3

Question 3: What are the consequences of using the vaccine in combination with other vaccines?

If you decide to vaccinate your child, the Hib vaccine needs to be given early in infancy when the risk is greatest, and to meet the requirements for day care and preschool. Avoiding more than one other shot at the same office visit can help reduce the risk of overload. The last injection is recommended at 12 to 15 months, so picking a different time than the MMR and chickenpox shots recommended during the same window would be wise.

Score: -3

Question 4: Are there ways to protect against the disease without getting the vaccine?

Antibiotics can treat the disease. According to the New York State Health Department: "Antibiotics, such as cefotaxime, ceftriaxone, or ampicillin with chloramphenicol, are generally used to treat serious infections. Rifampin is used in some circumstances as preventive treatment for persons who have been exposed to Hib disease."

Score: -2

OVERALL REWARD-RISK RATING: +1

The Big Picture: When Good Bugs Go Bad

We're conditioned to think of bacteria as bad things, a problem to human health. But most of us don't know that the human body contains over ten times more bacterial cells than human cells. Most of these are in our guts, but the "human microbiome" exists in every nook and cranny of our bodies and is essential to human health. Some of these are recognized as important enough that they're provided as supplements, or "probiotics." Natural-health nostrums tell us we can't get enough of germs like *Lactobacillus acidophilus* and *Bifidobacterium longum.*

Oddly, however, a number of the bacteria that hang around peacefully in our bodies can turn on us unexpectedly. The *Haemophilus influenza* B bacterium is one of these. It's present in the normal microbiome, especially in our sinus cavities and lungs. Every once in a while, and largely in infants, it can stop doing the (presumably good) things that put it in our bodies in the first place and start doing things it shouldn't. What is it that causes it to enter the brain and create meningitis in babies? No one knows. So in the absence of knowing what causes a good bug to turn bad, modern medicine has decided to kill it off entirely. Who knows what unintended consequence for our overall microbial health that campaign might create?

There are other bugs like this. The *streptococcus pneumonia* bacterium hangs out in similar places (the upper-respiratory tract), can go wrong in similar ways (meningitis and pneumonia), and has been targeted with vaccines (Prevnar 13®). Ditto for *Neisseria meningitides,* just substitute Menactra® for Prevnar inside the last parentheses.

There are other microbes with which we've been in harmony for centuries that have turned harmful unexpectedly. Poliovirus was pervasive in our environment until something changed in the late-nineteenth century that created frightening epidemics of paralytic poliomyelitis. What was the change? The well-known bacterium that caused the black plague, *Yersinia pestis*, killed millions during the Middle Ages. Today it's still around, but mostly threatens rodents in remote locations. Do we really know why?

We have become increasingly aware of the dangers of mass assault on our microbiome through overuse of antibiotics. But in the zeal to fight human illness with vaccine technologies, it appears we have lost sight of some of our more subtle vulnerabilities as well. Why do otherwise benign microbes turn virulent? What co-factors are we failing to recognize (especially pesticides) that might be more appropriate targets for disease prevention? What havoc might we wreak on the complex ecology of our friendly bugs when we single out one or more of them for attack?

Pneumococcal

Prevnar 13®, a vaccine to prevent bacterial meningitis and other illnesses, is recommended at 2, 4, 6, and 12–15 months. While the Hib vaccine is a "requirement" for preschool and day care in all but five states, the pneumococcal vaccine is only required in thirty-two. Like the Hib vaccine, it's not required for kindergarten and beyond because by then the risk of infection has all but passed. (In August 2014, the CDC's advisory committee recommended Prevnar 13® for adults over 65, setting off a predictable wave of lucrative TV advertising aimed at older adults.)

In commercial terms, the Prevnar brand, which was introduced by Wyeth (now Pfizer) in 2000, is the most successful vaccine ever launched, generating $31 billion since its inception. In its tenth year, it reached roughly $3 billion in worldwide revenues and has been generating about $4 billion a year since 2011. Its blockbuster status was a major reason Pfizer decided to buy the whole company that made it.

For any vaccine developer looking to maximize profits, Prevnar 13® sets the standard. It was adopted rapidly, both in the United States and globally; it has no competitors in its category; with the exception of one episode of supply problems in 2003, its growth has been continuous; and its history has been remarkably free of any reputation problems due to safety concerns.

The cloud hovering above this cheerful vista is a rather large one—the vaccine doesn't work very well, if at all, at actually preventing dangerous pneumococcal infections as a group. If you knock down seven strains of bacterium, as the original Prevnar did, a host of new ones can rise in their place, which is why the original seven-strain version was replaced with Prevnar 13®, with more in the pipeline. After many years and many billions of dollars, it's not at all clear that the vaccine has done much to reduce the worst forms of pneumococcal disease.

A recent study from Massachusetts on its effectiveness suggests that Prevnar, contrary to all expectations, did not reduce the incidence of invasive pneumococcal disease (IPD) in the state. Instead, although the forms of IPD caused by strains in the vaccine went down after Prevnar's introduction, IPD cases caused by other strains (some of which were even more dangerous than the original strains) rose almost immediately and in opposite proportions, to keep the rate of IPD in Massachusetts constant.

In plain language, the first version of Prevnar, the most commercially valuable vaccine in history, created no health benefits whatsoever. The jury is still out on Prevnar 13. We can't help but wonder when we'll be seeing Prevnar 29!

Reward Factors

Question 1: How bad is the disease?

The CDC says *Streptococcus pneumoniae* bacteria, or pneumococcus, can trigger many kinds of illness, from its namesake, severe pneumonia, to ear and sinus infections, to the blood infection known as bacteremia. It's called Invasive Pneumococcal Disease, because "it invades parts of the body that are normally free from germs," the CDC says.

Among the worst outcomes is meningitis, which inflames tissues and fluids around the brain and spinal cord.

Score: +4

Question 2: Does getting the vaccine help protect others from getting the same illness?

Pneumococcal disease is responsible for about 15 percent of all bacterial meningitis. But that percentage can be misleading, since vaccination doesn't protect against all of that 15 percent. These are pervasive bacteria, and since there are so many different strains of *Streptococcus pneumoniae,* getting the vaccine against 7 or 13 strains won't do much in terms of protecting against other strains.

Score: +1

Question 3: What is the risk of infection?

Really low, about one case in 100,000, the CDC says. Of those who contract the disease, about 1 in 10 die, which means the death rate is one in a million in the general population, higher in infants—about 1 in 10,000—and the elderly.

Score: +1

Question 4: How well does the vaccine work?

Because there are so many strains, it's hard to know how thorough the protection is against any specific strain; when the vaccine fails to protect against IPD, was that because vaccine strains or non-vaccine strains caused the infection? To date, it has the worst profile of the meningococcal vaccines, and its overall efficacy is questionable.

Score: +1

Risk Factors

Question 1: What are the vaccine's side effects?

The CDC says about half of those who get the vaccine have mild side effects, including redness or pain at the injection site. Fewer than one percent develop a fever, muscle aches, or more serious, local reactions. Allergic reactions are rare, but could include hives, swelling, breathing problems, or rapid heartbeat.

Score: -1

Question 2: What are the risks of chronic/severe illness and death?

Despite its benign reputation, according to Gayle DeLong's analysis it has one of the worst safety records for serious, adverse events and one of the worst risk/benefit profiles. The rate of serious injury or death from IPD in 1999, the year before the vaccine was introduced, was 1 in 100,000; by contrast, the rate of serious, reported adverse events, including 649 deaths, in the years since the vaccine has been given was 1 in 25,000.

Score: -3

Question 3: What are the consequences of using the vaccine in combination with other vaccines?

Like the Hib vaccine, it's also worth getting for children only during infancy and toddlerhood, and on the same schedule as the Hib vaccine of 2, 4, 6, and 15–18 months. If you decide to use this vaccine, you could consider staggering it to avoid other shots.

Score: -3

Question 4: Are there ways to protect against the disease without getting the vaccine?

Antibiotics can treat the disease. According to the CDC's Pink Book, "Resistance to penicillin and other antibiotics is common . . . so treatment will usually include broad-spectrum antibiotics like cephalosporin and vancomycin."

Score: -2

OVERALL REWARD-RISK RATING: -2

Meningococcal

Meningococcal meningitis is a terrible disease that causes horrifying headlines:

- "Killer at College: Meningitis threatens students" —NBC.

- "Final test results have confirmed that a Georgetown University student died from bacterial meningitis, school officials said Thursday night," —WJLA TV, Washington.

- "At the University of California at Santa Barbara, where a fourth bacterial meningitis case was confirmed this week, a freshman lacrosse player had both feet amputated. Campus leaders have suspended fraternity parties and other social events and ramped up cleaning in residence halls and recreation facilities." —Washington Post.

- "Princeton University will administer another round of meningitis vaccines next week as U.S. health and university officials confirmed that the Drexel University student who died earlier this month had the same rare strain that sickened several people at Princeton last year." —NJ.com

In the face of such terrible and tragic facts, is there even an argument about whether the meningococcal vaccine is a good idea? Yes, there is.

It's not the severity of the disease, which is indisputable, but the rarity that puts this vaccine on the minus side of our Reward-Risk Rating. That doesn't lessen the tragic consequences of the disease, but it does mean you need to decide if the vaccine is worth it for your family.

The disease appears to thrive in cramped quarters like boarding schools, barracks, and colleges. The rate for college freshmen is 1 in 63,000—a total of 36 cases in over 2 million freshman.

So in the worst case of all, the risk of death from the illness is 10 percent, or 1 in 630,000, fewer than 5 deaths per year. Compare that again to another unlikely event—getting hit by lightning. The risk of bacterial meningitis in general is higher than, but on the order of, a lightning strike.

If all meningitis came from a single bacterium, then maybe a vaccine strategy would be stronger. The problems is, there are at least dozens of different bacteria involved, and each individual vaccine only protects against a narrow range. So each vaccination choice balances the risk of an adverse event with an exceedingly rare chance of meaningful protection.

Another problem is that, as everyone acknowledges, vaccines are unavoidably unsafe. With meningitis itself a low-probability event, what are the probabilities of serious effects from the vaccine?

Reward Factors

Question 1: How bad is the disease?

Meningitis is a very dangerous illness and can cause lifelong disability and death. Frequent news reports about students bring home the sad consequences.

Score: +3

Question 2: Does getting the vaccine help protect others from getting the same illness?

Yes, it appears to protect the spread of certain strains of meningitis, which is why so many colleges require it at least for those living in dormitories. One problem, however, is that (like Prevnar®) the approved meningococcal vaccine, Menactra®, protects against a limited number of strains, in this case four. The meningitis scare at Princeton described above involved a meningococcal strain that wasn't present in Menactra®. Urgent efforts to offer vaccines to concerned students required bringing in an unlicensed vaccine from Europe, one that protected against a strain that isn't included in Menactra®, serogroup B.

Score: +1

Question 3: What is the risk of infection?

As we've noted above: very, very low. Freshmen in college dormitories have seemed to be the highest-risk group, and even in this group the risk of infection is extremely low.

Score: 0

Question 4: How well does the vaccine work?

It appears to be effective—only two doses are recommended. But again, since the occurrence of infection is so low, how does one really know whether the vaccine has been helping or not? Or if other strains of meningococcus might arise in place of the vaccine strains.

Score: +2

Risk Factors

Question 1: What are the vaccine's side effects?

Adolescents, for whom the vaccine is targeted, can experience fainting or seizure-like spells after vaccination. Half of those who get the shot have mild side effects like redness or pain, and a small percentage develop mild fever.

Score: -1

Question 2: What are the risks of chronic/severe illness and death?

Serious reactions are very rare, the CDC says. But data compiled by Gayle DeLong shows 24 deaths and 167 serious, adverse events reported to VAERS, a rate of 5 per million. Because the rate of infection is so low, this is another vaccine where in DeLong's analysis the risks outweigh the benefits—in this case the risks are five times higher.

Score: -2

Question 3: What are the consequences of using the vaccine in combination with other vaccines?

The vaccine generally is not given at the same time as other shots. If that issue comes up, it would be wise to separate them as there is no major lineup of vaccines at the age it's recommended. VAERS reports have indicated especially bad interactions with Gardasil®, the HPV vaccine, including convulsions, seizures, spontaneous abortions, and Guillain-Barré Syndrome. Parents can and should ask for it to be given on a separate visit from any other shots the child might be due to receive.

Score: -1

Question 4: Are there ways to protect against the disease without getting the vaccine?

Avoid crowded living conditions and dubious hygiene; live in off-campus housing or in less-cramped rooms. That is not always possible for college students.

Score: -2

OVERALL REWARD-RISK RATING: 0

Part III:
What You Can Do

CHAPTER 12

CHOOSING THE RIGHT PATH FOR YOUR FAMILY

NOW THAT WE'VE TAKEN THE CDC'S CHILDHOOD-vaccine schedule apart, perhaps in more ways than one, this section will help you put it together to fit your family's needs. Making the right choices about vaccinating your children is not an easy one and involves both individual choices and an overall plan: what are your own beliefs about what is best for your child? What are the local rules and mandates in your state that you will face? How do you want to work with your pediatrician or other health-service providers? How do you want to work with day care services and the school system? Ultimately, what is the overall vaccination schedule you want to choose for your child?

Some of our friends are against vaccination on principle; we are not, but we respect their position. Like them, we support choice as the bedrock of health freedom, but that choice includes the freedom to vaccinate, and a lot of parents are going to choose to vaccinate. They should not be left without unbiased information on how to provide the vaccines they choose to give their own children.

So the first thing to understand is this truly is *your* choice—not ours (we're not recommending any specific schedule here), not any one doctor's, and certainly not the government's. This is America, after all, the land of the free and the home of the brave—which you'll need to be as you think and act for yourselves about this fraught topic. It's impossible to avoid hearing dire talk about "requirements," "firing" parents from medical practices, or expelling kids from school if they don't follow the letter of the federal-vaccine chart.

But as citizens, we still hold the keys to choices affecting our off-spring, and we do not hand them over to anybody in return for the right to a public education or any other inducement. The starting point for the discussion is freedom of speech and freedom of choice, and the fact that parents are in charge when it comes to decisions involving their children as long as those decisions don't hinder their health or wellbeing. Given the well-founded concerns we've demonstrated about individual vaccines—as well as the bloated childhood-immunization schedule—making careful vaccination choices hardly counts as jeopardizing kids' health. In fact, the real threat is not stepping out of line but mindlessly toeing it, at least when your child's wellbeing is at stake.

When we speak of vaccination "mandates," what we are really talking about begins as a series of *recommendations* by the CDC's Advisory Committee on Immunization Practices (itself an oddly constructed, unaccountable, and highly conflicted group, many of whom have financial ties to the pharmaceutical business). These recommendations are routinely adopted by the CDC and by national medical associations. State governments then consult the list before deciding which to require for public school admission or access to day care centers.

"There are no federal vaccination laws," acknowledges the pro-vaccine group, A Shot of Prevention. "However, just as the government requires immunizations for those who volunteer to join the military, and health providers may require employees to be vaccinated in a medical setting, immunization requirements for public school enrollment are determined by individual states. Parents are not forced to vaccinate their children. Rather, they're given a choice as to whether they want their children to attend public school and therefore be vaccinated according to state admission policies."

Of course, those states allow exemptions of various kinds and degree as part of their "admission policies," which we'll get to in a moment. First, it's quite revealing how much these vaccine "mandates" vary by state—to the point that several vaccines you might be pressured to get by your pediatrician have no bearing on your child's school attendance. A common set of vaccines is almost always required for kindergarten, usually the DTaP, MMR, hep B, polio, and chicken pox vaccines—all but the hep B and chicken pox vaccines predating the lifting of liability on vaccine manufacturers in 1986. But not all of today's 16 CDC-recommended vaccines are mandated for school—not by a long shot. (See chart on next page based on data from the National Network for Immunization Information.)

Take the authors' home states. Dan lives in Virginia. For kindergarteners, the required vaccines are DTaP, MMR, polio, chicken pox and hep B. Those shots plus the Hib and pneumococcal vaccines are required for children in day care. The HPV shot is mandated for girls starting in the sixth grade. The meningococcal vaccine is required for college.

Massachusetts, Mark's home state, has the same kindergarten requirements, but no pneumococcal-vaccine requirement for preschool and no HPV mandate for sixth-grade girls. (Virginia, in fact, is the *only* state to require the HPV vaccine for school—along with the District of Columbia—but there's an easy opt-out. And even Virginia doesn't require it for boys, despite the CDC recommendation that all children receive it.) Massachusetts requires the meningococcal vaccine for boarding school students in seventh grade, but among college students, only freshmen who live on campus.

Seriously, folks: How crucial are hep A, influenza, rotavirus, pneumococcal, meningococcal, and HPV vaccines if Virginia and Massachusetts either don't require them at all (hep A, influenza, and rotavirus vaccines), don't conform on which ones they do require (pneumococcal and HPV), don't agree on who needs them when (meningococcal), or don't require them unless your child goes to preschool (pneumococcal and Hib). These are all FDA-approved, CDC-recommended childhood vaccines that the American Academy of Pediatrics says all children should get on a precise schedule. What's the matter with state government in Virginia and Massachusetts—are they founts of dangerous anti-vaccine quackery?

No, they're not, and neither are parents who likewise consider the CDC recommendations, and proceed to make their own choices.

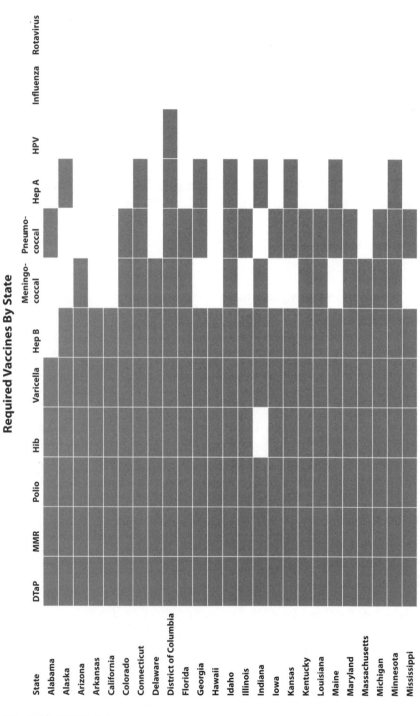

Required Vaccines By State

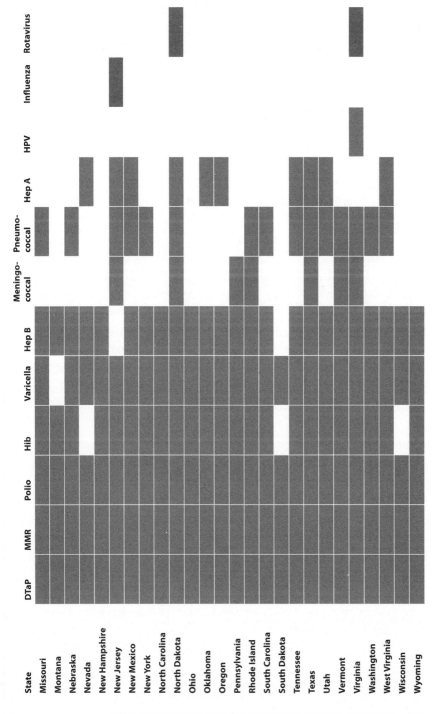

Careful parents just want to prevent both serious illness and serious vaccine injury, protect their autonomy, and keep medical interventions to a minimum. We've talked and corresponded with hundreds of parents over the years on these issues and have encountered as many choices as there are questions. We've learned that there are numerous different and legitimate routes to balancing these concerns. Here are three very different but very consistent models we've seen.

Model One: Opt Out. For those who are opposed to vaccination and don't trust any vaccines, there is a comprehensive approach and a clear recourse: choose homeschooling or sympathetic private schools over the preschool and public school system and its associated mandates, avoid mainstream pediatric doctors, and partner with naturopathic medical providers instead. In the absence of the pressure of conventional pediatrics and school attendance mandates, parents can choose not to vaccinate their children at all. Far from being an oddball decision, this path is followed by a large and supportive community of Americans who opt out of all vaccinations, period. The homeschool movement seems to be growing, and you can join it. In many states religious and personal belief exemptions are available (see below).

Model Two: Go Slow, Be Selective. For people who like to follow the rules, want to minimize any dissonance from family, friends, schools, and doctors, but are still concerned about vaccination risks and want to be extra careful in their approach, there are other options. You can be selective about vaccines you choose and the pace that you adopt. Avoid vaccines when you can avoid the risk of disease in other ways (for example, hep B), avoid the worst ones with little cost to you or little benefit, avoid the ones that aren't required for school and that other nations or states don't recommend. (If preventing chicken pox is so critical, why isn't it recommended in Britain or Nevada?) Of the remaining set that you want your child to receive, you can adopt a more relaxed schedule, delaying and spreading out each procedure.

Model 3: Minimize Risky Interventions. For people who are deeply concerned about vaccination risk, who don't trust the system, but don't want to go all the way to the point of not vaccinating at all and simply want to choose a minimalist vaccination schedule (one that makes vaccination for their children "safe, voluntary, and rare"), there is yet another course. You can exercise your right to a philosophical or religious exemption where available and avoid even some vaccines that schools require. You can choose only those vaccines that protect against diseases that present the largest risk to your infant, such as early pertussis, or to another mother's developing fetus, such as congenital rubella. This minimalist list might also be administered with fewer boosters and at more carefully targeted points in development when the risk of damage to the developing brain, gut, and immune system is lower.

Availability of Vaccine Exemptions by State

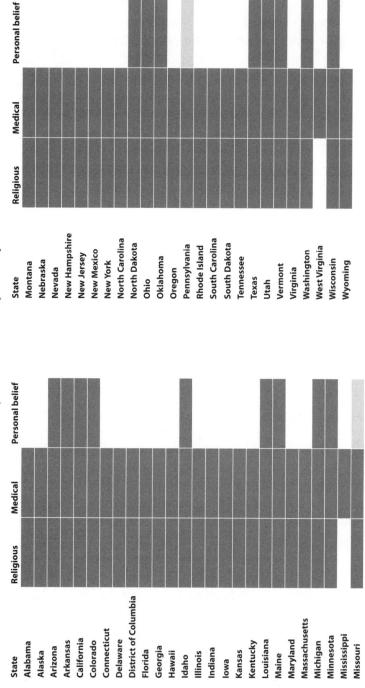

Missouri allows personal belief exemptions for day care, preschool, and nursery school only.

Pennsylvania personal belief exemptions allowed on the basis of a strong moral or ethical conviction similar to a religious belief.

CHAPTER 13

CONSIDERING THE ALTERNATIVES

LET'S START BY EXPLORING THE MIDDLE GROUND with a thoughtful approach developed in the medical practice of Dr. Elizabeth Mumper, whom we introduced in Part 1. A mainstream, respected pediatrician for thirty years in Lynchburg, Virginia, she became concerned the soaring vaccine schedule might be one of the factors contributing to the rise of immune and neurological disorders in her practice—with outcomes as seemingly different as juvenile diabetes, asthma, allergies, attention disorders, and autism.

So Mumper decided to create her own, modified-vaccination schedule, one that would meet the requirements for preschool and public school attendance in Virginia but give her more opportunity to monitor infants *as individuals* and to watch for negative consequences of particular shots. (Mumper notes: "My schedule is a starting point and may be delayed or modified by the parents.")

"I developed my vaccine schedule after listening to 400 or 500 stories directly from parents who thought that the health of their children changed after particular vaccines in particular circumstances. Many of the kids affected were in the autism spectrum but not necessarily, because sometimes the children seemed to have immune dysregulation but not neurologic dysfunction which parents suspected were related in some way to vaccines," Mumper explained to us.

"So I looked at the Virginia vaccine schedule and tried to figure out how I could construct something that would eliminate at least some of the triggers that I thought I was hearing from the parents, but walk the line of not having parents end up in legal trouble or their kids suspended from school."

She was guided by another principle: "The most crucial time to be making good vaccine decisions is when the baby is very young, when their immune system hasn't declared itself yet and when we are not sure how well they are going to develop."

Mumper has published a scientific paper reporting on her approach; this is the revised schedule she proposes. She includes the day care-related Hib and Prevnar vaccines. Her schedule has no shots before two months of age, no more than two shots at a time, and at least one month between visits. Yet her patients easily meet school requirements. (At twelve months she discusses the chicken pox vaccine with parents; at two or three years, hep B; and at the kindergarten physical, follow-up DTaP, polio, MMR, and chicken pox shots, all listed for school admission.)

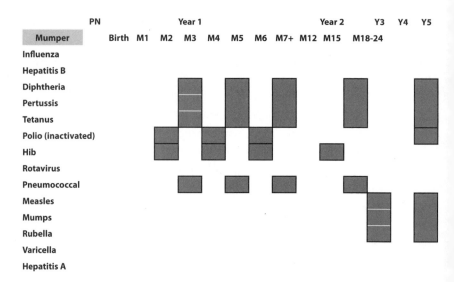

The most immediate difference from the CDC schedule is the absence of the hep B vaccine at birth. "The first thing that struck me," Mumper said, "was the lack of logic in giving the hepatitis B vaccine to all babies. In my community I always know the hep B status of my moms. I counsel them (if hep B negative) to politely decline it.

First, nurses would come back to them and say, are you sure? The nurses were trying to do their job. Over time, if these people are my patients, the nurses no longer argue with the new mothers.

"Unless it's somebody new to the area, I pretty much have 100 percent no hep B vaccination in my practice in early infancy unless the mother is hepatitis B positive."

She feels the opposite about Hib. "I personally love the Hib vaccine and I think it's very low risk. When I was an intern over thirty years ago now, I have vivid memories of previously normal beautiful babies coming in with haemophilus meningitis. I would do their spinal tap, and pus would hit me in the chest, the cerebrospinal fluid was under such pressure. Even though I see babies who get a little bit of fever or puffiness after the shot, I don't see Hib vaccine as having a high potential for neurologic damage."

The key for Mumper is being alert to the overall health and development of the child. She's particularly cautious with children born by C-section; who got antibiotics or were in neonatal-intensive care as infants; have eczema, indicating autoimmunity; are unusually fussy; or aren't smiling back at their parents at four to six weeks. "Those are the babies I might have a question mark in my mind about either their neurologic status or their immune status, and I would say maybe we would not start vaccines at two months or we would just give one vaccine at a time.

"I'm sure I make some judgment calls that are right and some that are wrong every day, but the big thing for me is to not just follow a cookbook but follow the individual child's risk versus benefit, which is how we're supposed to make decisions about drugs. But somehow when we give the medicinal agent as a vaccine, individual decision making goes by the wayside in favor of one size fits all public health vaccine schedules."

She gives the MMR vaccine at age two, not at twelve months. "I don't do MMR at a year of age. I've heard way too many stories about regression after MMR that was given when children were sick or in conjunction with Varivax [the chicken pox vaccine]. I do not give MMR if a child has recently had antibiotics within 4 to 6 weeks, has diarrhea or inflammatory bowel symptoms, or has recently been sick." The vaccination schedule, in other words, bends to the welfare of the individual child, not the other way around.

Perhaps the best-known alternative schedule is Dr. Bob Sears'. He offers several variations; "Dr. Bob's Complete Alternative Vaccine Schedule" differs from Mumper's in several ways, such as the inclusion of rotavirus and influenza vaccines; MMR at the standard 12 months; hep B at a delayed 2 years, 6 months; as well as HPV at 13 to 14 years rather than the recommended 11 to 12. Mumper, who questions that vaccine's effectiveness and is concerned about reports of severe injury, has never given it. The vaccine is available at the Health Department for those who choose it.

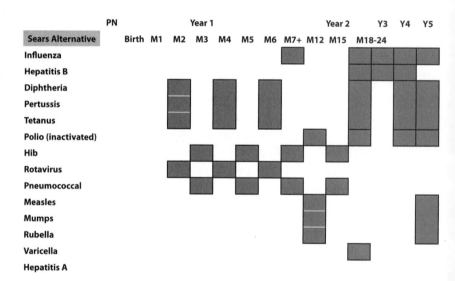

Sears has taken a lot of flak from the mainstream-pediatric establishment for this detour from the straight-and-narrow vaccination schedule. *Pediatrics* published an article in 2007 titled, "The Problem With Dr. Bob's Alternative Vaccine Schedule" and concluded Sears misrepresents vaccine science and "misinforms parents trying to make the right decisions for their children."

Many vaccine-safety advocates, on the other hand, fear that Dr. Sears' featured approach includes far too many CDC-recommended vaccines. To his credit, however, he presents other, less-aggressive options as well. "Dr. Bob's Selective Vaccine Schedule" offers fewer vaccines than his complete alternative schedule; it, too, includes the rotavirus vaccine but skips the MMR, chicken pox, flu, and hep B shots before age ten. He also suggests delayed versions of those schedules, with no vaccines before six months, before one year, and before two years.

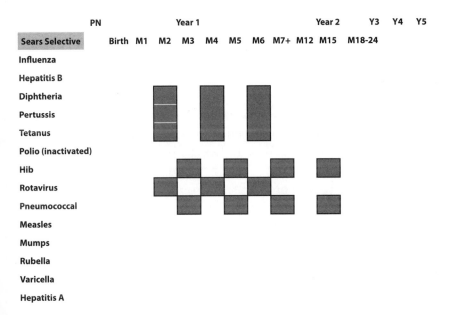

Sears Selective	PN		Year 1							Year 2		Y3	Y4	Y5
	Birth	M1	M2	M3	M4	M5	M6	M7+	M12	M15	M18-24			
Influenza														
Hepatitis B														
Diphtheria				■		■		■						
Pertussis				■		■		■						
Tetanus				■		■		■						
Polio (inactivated)														
Hib				■		■		■		■				
Rotavirus			■		■		■							
Pneumococcal				■		■		■		■				
Measles														
Mumps														
Rubella														
Varicella														
Hepatitis A														

Based on our own Reward-Risk Rating, if you like Dr. Sears' approach but prefer to be a bit more selective in how you vaccinate your child, the rotavirus and flu shots could fall off your list in the first round—they each got negative ratings on our scale as both unnecessary and higher risk—and the MMR could be postponed. It has been associated with autistic regression and bowel disease when given at twelve months.

Sears, perhaps mindful of his high-profile position as one of the few pediatricians to challenge vaccine orthodoxy, expresses less conviction than we do about the risks of autism from vaccines. "Overall, I agree that the majority of the mainstream research does not show a link between vaccines and autism," he writes. He goes on to criticize conflicts of interest on both sides of the vaccine-autism debate.

Citing rulings by the vaccine "court," he concludes: "What is very clear, however, is that vaccines have triggered autism in a very small number of children. A phrase I recently heard sums it up very well: Vaccines don't cause autism . . . except when they do."

At least Sears acknowledges a link, but in our view it may leave parents less concerned than they should be. To us, the evidence is clear: Vaccines have triggered autism in a *large* number of children. This may be an instance where not being medical professionals makes it easier for people like us to tell the truth about *iatrogenic* (i.e. medically induced) injury.

As Mumper says of resistance she's encountered to any change to the vaccine regimen, like delaying hep B vaccines from the day of birth, "Even though doctors would like to think we're very rational, we're also emotional and human beings. No pediatrician goes into medicine to try to hurt babies. So when you have to face the fact that you've given thousands of vaccines in your career and you've probably hurt a few kids neurologically, that is not an easy thing to accept."

Privately, she says, some doctors have e-mailed her to ask about postponing the hep B vaccine. Our advice: Don't wait for the rest of the medical profession to catch up to her cautious, common-sense approach.

What, then, would be better than the current vaccine schedule? The short answer is almost anything—any carefully selected schedule, starting with Mumper's and Sears', with fewer vaccines in the critical first few months of life. Another logical place to look for alternatives: *before* the deluge—before the vaccine liability protection act of 1986 led to so many more vaccines and, we believe, contributed directly to the soaring rates of autism, ADHD, juvenile diabetes, bipolar, asthma, and much more.

Amazingly, given that American children were healthier then than now (see Part I), just seven vaccines were recommended— the DPT shot, the live-polio vaccine, and the MMR shot. While these undoubtedly had serious side effects in some children—the pertussis vaccine caused brain damage that led to a safer acellular version, the DTaP vaccine—the vaccine schedule in place back then clearly was not causing the array of adverse events we see today.

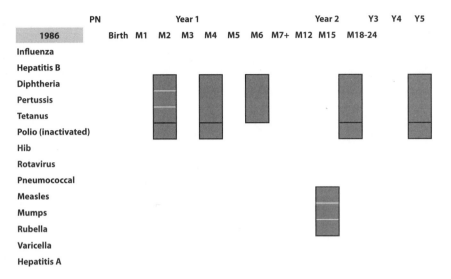

1986	PN		Year 1						Year 2		Y3	Y4	Y5
	Birth	M1	M2	M3	M4	M5	M6	M7+	M12	M15	M18-24		
Influenza													
Hepatitis B													
Diphtheria													
Pertussis													
Tetanus													
Polio (inactivated)													
Hib													
Rotavirus													
Pneumococcal													
Measles													
Mumps													
Rubella													
Varicella													
Hepatitis A													

Generation Rescue, an autism-advocacy group, has proposed returning to that schedule until conclusive research is done on the individual and combined effects of today's vaccination regime.

But for those who carry the legitimate concern that even before The National Childhood Vaccine Injury Act of 1986, there were too many vaccine injuries, there's a refinement to the Generation Rescue model that would be more cautious still.

Like Mumper, we have concerns about giving the MMR vaccine at twelve months. So you could move it even later than age two to age three, just past the thirty-six months mark for an autism diagnosis. There is little evidence that the MMR vaccine *alone*—absent the onslaught of other shots and the mercury-preservative, thimerosal—has caused high rates of autism, especially when given later. (As we pointed out in Part I, CDC senior scientist William Thompson has accused the agency of hiding an elevated risk of autism in black males who got the MMR vaccine before thirty-six months.)

You could move the first DTaP shot from two months to three months, in light of the research that showed earlier vaccination increased the risk of asthma substantially, while also protecting your infant against increasingly common pertussis infection.

And you could get your child's titers—which measure the level of antibodies to the disease circulating in the·blood—checked after both the MMR and the DTaP shots to see if one dose had conferred immunity, making follow-up shots unnecessary. For a couple of hundred dollars (unfortunately, insurance doesn't normally cover this), the risk of reaction from follow-up shots could be eliminated in the majority of cases. DTaP vaccine reactions are known to be more severe in later shots in the series.

Call this model the One-Three-Three Alternative Schedule: one DTaP shot at three months, then check for titers; one MMR shot at three years, then check for titers. Only if the titers showed the vaccine had not taken hold would you consider boosters.

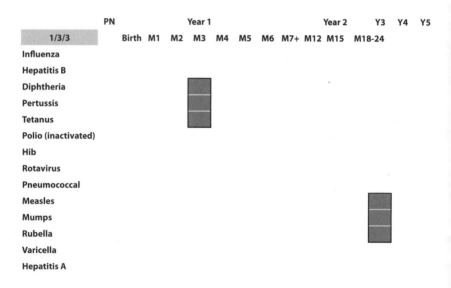

1/3/3	PN			Year 1						Year 2		Y3	Y4	Y5
	Birth	M1	M2	M3	M4	M5	M6	M7+	M12	M15	M18-24			
Influenza														
Hepatitis B														
Diphtheria														
Pertussis														
Tetanus														
Polio (inactivated)														
Hib														
Rotavirus														
Pneumococcal														
Measles														
Mumps														
Rubella														
Varicella														
Hepatitis A														

Because these are combination shots—and the MMR is three live viruses—the case for each component of each shot is necessarily mixed. As we discussed in Part II, the rubella vaccine may be the best immunization ever invented. It prevents a real tragedy—fetal death or grievous damage if a pregnant woman catches the otherwise benign disease. If one were to make a case for the value of getting a vaccine for the greater good, this would be it.

Unfortunately, rubella is attached to the hydra-headed MMR vaccine; we share the concern of researchers who believe that just putting the viruses together in one shot raises the risk of adverse events due to viral interference, as we discussed in Part II. What's more, the mumps portion may be the single *dumbest* vaccine as currently constituted, for a disease with very few serious consequences when caught in childhood, now pushed into later and more dangerous ages by the failure (and alleged cover-up of the failure) of the vaccine itself.

There's more of a case for the measles vaccine than for the mumps vaccine, because measles can have rare, serious, and even fatal consequences, though mostly where poor nutrition and sanitation prevail. Dr. Andrew Wakefield, who raised the initial alarm about regressive autism and bowel disease following the MMR vaccine, still recommended the shots be given individually a year apart while the safety of the combined vaccine was assessed, and he vaccinated his own children.

A truly important public health measure, we believe, would be to bring back separate measles, mumps, and rubella shots. In the past, these were available, but Merck, the sole manufacturer licensed to market the MMR vaccine in the US, stopped making them. Offering that choice again—and choice is the heart of the issue—would probably increase vaccine uptake and decrease measles outbreaks.

As for the DTaP vaccine: Pertussis—popularly known as whooping cough—does remain a risk, apparently because the new acellular vaccine appears to either fail outright or wear off quickly, thereby weakening its role in the fight against the current strain of the disease. Whooping cough is worth preventing, especially in infants, and we give the stand-alone pertussis component our highest Reward-Risk Rating. Diphtheria, on the other hand, is virtually extinct; there have been fewer than five cases reported in the last ten years, the CDC says. Some believe the diphtheria vaccine is still part of the DTaP shot mainly to act as an immune booster for the pertussis component. Regarding tetanus, the disease is now rarely encountered, and the risk is treatable with a tetanus-immune globulin injection (and possibly vaccination) at the time of exposure; a routine, lifelong vaccine regimen seems superfluous.

The MMR and DTaP vaccines, remember, are universally required by states for school admission, so a child who gets them is already partway through the schoolhouse door.

While polio—another universally mandated vaccine for school admission—has a fearsome history, the vaccine hardly seems necessary now unless someone is planning to visit certain parts of the developing world. Essential to wiping out polio epidemics in the United States when it was introduced in the 1950s, it has dubious value in modern-day America. "Some patients opt out of giving their babies polio vaccines early, but we do recommend the series. We discuss that the likelihood of an infant getting polio in the US approaches zero," Mumper told us. "The rationale for continued polio vaccine is a public health issue. We struggle with the balance between individual health vs. public health."

Put bluntly, Bill Gates—who has committed nearly $2 billion to a worldwide-eradication campaign, may want you to get the polio vaccine until his role in history is secure; your two-month-old infant doesn't need it.

CHAPTER 14

THE NO-VACCINES OPTION

BEYOND THESE ALTERNATIVES LIES THE NO-VACCINES OPTION. This option is championed by an increasing number of natural-health advocates as well as parents who have witnessed vaccine damage (and the subsequent denial of injury and compensation by doctors and the government). Many believe the process of tinkering with the immune system *always* results in an unnatural and damaging outcome, and the case that vaccines wiped out diseases like polio and even smallpox is simply not convincing.

Laura Hayes, whose son has autism caused by vaccine reactions, pulled those threads together when she wrote on our blog:

"I still think it is of paramount importance for people to understand that the term 'safe vaccines' is an oxymoron, and therefore, I would not agree that there is any 'smart approach to vaccination.'

"By their very nature, vaccines cannot be made safe, as they artificially and unnaturally stimulate the immune system (by injecting these toxic cocktails, versus inhaling or consuming them, the first part of the immune system's response is bypassed, which is essential to trigger the next parts of the immune response).

"Then, multiply that unsafe effect by giving multiple vaccines at once, without consideration of family history or body weight, and before any allergies or metabolic problems have been discerned, and that is a recipe for absolute disaster.

"Informed consent with regards to vaccines is also compromised, making it impossible to implement, because our own government agencies have been extremely busy covering up inconvenient truths for a number of decades now. This cover-up includes the fact that the toxic amounts of thimerosal in vaccines from the late 1980s through the early 2000s (and today, thanks to flu vaccines, and vaccines with 'trace amounts'... who do you really think is monitoring such things?) was highly statistically linked to autism, not to mention to a host of other debilitating childhood epidemics we were and still are witnessing in our children in this country.

"I think that we as a community of people who have either personally experienced vaccine injury/death, and/or who have seen our children and loved ones experience it, must continue to shed light on all of the aforementioned issues. Personally, I have no problem being called anti-vaccine, because I am. I think vaccination is a barbaric practice that is not founded on any sound science, and as a matter of fact, we now have mountains of evidence showing us that it is a practice we should immediately halt."

Asked to read a draft of our book, Hayes says we have been far too generous in our vaccine ratings section, erring in favor of rating vaccines too highly. She contends that in reality, there is no way to accurately rate any vaccine:

"Since the vaccine 'safety' and 'efficacy' studies have not been performed in a scientifically valid manner (as we have discussed) or reported in an ethical and honest manner (as admitted by recent whistleblowers, and as has been uncovered by parents and others over the years via FOIA requests and other means), there is no basis for any type of vaccine claim, other than that they have harmed and killed.

"In the absence of proper vaccine studies, both of individual vaccines and of the vaccine schedule as it is recommended to be given, and in the absence of a comparative study of the vaccinated versus the unvaccinated," she argues, "any claims of safety or efficacy, and any ratings of vaccines, are not only premature, they can't be done at this point in time." It is a point of view we respect.

Clearly, the never-vaccinated contingent is growing in the United States, and there is mounting evidence that never-vaccinated kids may well be healthier than their fully vaccinated counterparts.

- Among the Amish, who often don't vaccinate or do so selectively, autism in the absence of genetic disorders to which they are prone appears to be strikingly rare. Dr. Heng Wang told us in 2005 that among 10,000 Amish kids he has seen in northeastern Ohio, only one had autism, and that child was vaccinated. We found just one case among the Amish of a previously typical child with regressive autism; she had been removed from her family at age two by medical authorities in a dispute over her health care, fully vaccinated during that period, and returned at age three with full-syndrome autism. The prevalence of asthma and Alzheimer's is also much lower in the Amish.

- Medical practices that accept parents who choose not to follow the CDC schedule, or not vaccinate at all, report much lower rates of chronic disorders. Elizabeth Mumper's practice in Virginia has had only one case of autism out of hundreds of new patients since she revised her approach around 2000, and no new cases of juvenile diabetes. Dr. Mayer Eisenstein's Homefirst Medical Services in Chicago has treated upwards of 50,000 never-vaccinated children, and according to Eisenstein there have been zero cases of autism and virtually no asthma in that population. Despite the attention our reporting on Homefirst in 2007 has generated, public health officials have not followed up.

- Surveys consistently find less autism and other disorders in never-vaccinated children. "We surveyed over 9,000 boys in California and Oregon and found that vaccinated boys had a 155% greater chance of having a neurological disorder like ADHD or autism than unvaccinated boys," Generation Rescue says.

- Even slight delays in vaccination appear to have significant results—putting off the first DTaP shot from the recommended two months to four months cut the asthma rate by more than half in one study. Getting the first DPT shot a few weeks *ahead of schedule* increased the asthma rate by 60 percent over those who got it at the recommended time. Even small adjustments can make a big difference.

- Never-vaccinated, homeschooled students appear to have lower rates of autism and other disorders. "There was this whole subculture of folks who went into homeschooling so they would never have to vaccinate their kids," Dr. Jeff Bradstreet told us. "In that subset, unless they were massively exposed to mercury through lots of amalgams (mercury dental fillings in the mother) and/or big-time fish eating, I've not had a single case." A formal "vax-unvax" study of homeschooled children funded in part by Generation Rescue and led by independent researchers at Jackson State University is under way.
- Members of Congress, intrigued by these observations, have repeatedly introduced bills to compel the National Institutes of Health to look at health outcomes in vaccinated versus never-vaccinated American children. The bills have not gotten any traction, amid bogus complaints that a prospective study would be unethical and a retrospective study would be impossible. No one is suggesting the former, and there is no reason the latter should be difficult, given the hundreds of thousands of never-vaccinated children in the United States.

Even within the confines of orthodox medicine, there is considerably more wiggle room on the vaccine "schedule" than a mainstream pediatrician would probably want you to know. The CDC provides a range of months during which many vaccinations can be given, and a "catch-up" schedule that tacitly acknowledges later vaccinations are nonetheless protective of personal and public health. The CDC's Parents Guide suggests taking "advantage of the age ranges for certain vaccine doses to customize your baby's personal immunization schedule, reducing the number of shots she gets at a given visit." (This at the same time the CDC tells doctors to use as many combination shots per visit as possible.)

With regard to families who choose not to vaccinate, hardline pediatricians are often proudly vocal about "firing their patients," because they don't want to bother with a cautious parent who actually wants to spend some time with their child's doctor obtaining their basic right to informed consent. The AAP, at least officially, suggests working with parents who refuse vaccination rather than kicking them out of the practice or calling in child protective services. "The problem of parental refusal of immunization for children is an important one for pediatricians," guidance published in its professional journal notes:

- "Many parents have concerns related to 1 or 2 specific vaccines. A useful strategy in working with families who refuse immunization is to discuss each vaccine separately. The benefits and risks of vaccines differ, and a parent who is reluctant to accept the administration of 1 vaccine may be willing to allow others.
- "In other cases, a parent may be willing to permit a schedule of immunization that does not require multiple injections at a single visit.
- "Families with doubts about immunization should still have access to good medical care, and maintaining the relationship in the face of disagreement conveys respect and at the same time allows the child access to medical care. Furthermore, a continuing relationship allows additional opportunity to discuss the issue of immunization over time.
- "Continued refusal after adequate discussion should be respected unless the child is put at significant risk of serious harm (as, for example, might be the case during an epidemic). Only then should state agencies be involved to override parental discretion on the basis of medical neglect."

"The benefits and risks of vaccines differ" and "continued refusal after adequate discussion should be respected"—you might want to copy that for your next well-baby visit.

We don't believe it's ever appropriate for pediatricians to pressure parents to forego vaccine choice or be "fired" from their medical practice, and there is no basis whatsoever for involving child welfare agencies in parental vaccine decisions, since there is no legal requirement to receive any of them.

Nonetheless, and despite these suggestions from the American Academy of Pediatrics itself, it happens all the time in pediatricians' offices across the country. When it does, parents either need to convince their doctor to follow their wishes, or they need to find another health care provider who will. As a commenter who calls herself "Nick's Mom" wrote on our blog:

"I had received a 'we're going to fire you from our practice if you don't vaccinate' notice in the mail. At first, I thought it was really scary, but then I realized I was in charge of our family's health services and that these doctors work for us! You should have seen the look on the nurse's face when I told her that her doctor's office practice of refusing medical care to children with vaccine injury history shows that they don't care about my children so I was going to go elsewhere for their medical treatment. We went to a general practitioner's office after that and never were harassed again about vaccines! GP's aren't beholden to the AAP either! It's such a feeling of freedom because I conquered that fear and my children are all better off from that decision."

CHAPTER 15

HOW TO
OPT OUT

ANOTHER STEP THAT PARENTS CAN TAKE is to secure exemptions from vaccination based on philosophical, religious, or medical grounds.

In Mississippi and West Virginia, only medical exemptions are allowed. This means parents must offer proof their children would suffer adverse consequences from vaccines due to a medical condition that the state recognizes as a risk. We'll discuss those risks—and others that we believe you should know about, even if health officials don't recognize them—in a moment.

All other states allow either philosophical or religious exemptions, or both. Several sources provide state-level specifics. The National Vaccine Information Center (NVIC.org) offers a fifty-state chart of exemptions. The CDC has a fifty-state interactive guide. The National Council of State Legislatures has a fifty-state list with links to the state-by-state statutes. (The NVIC site, in particular, is a trove of reliable and detailed information about vaccine requirements, exemptions, risks, and much more. It's worth consulting at length.)

Philosophical objections are the easiest to obtain and usually require only a written statement from the parents that their philosophical beliefs include opposition to all vaccines or to a particular one. Religious exemptions often (but not always) require that the family follows a recognized religion or adheres to a coherent religious-belief system that counsels against or forbids vaccination in general or a particular vaccine.

Let's take a look at the largest state, California, which allows all three exemptions—medical, religious, and philosophical. The devil is often in the details; the nature and availability of these exemptions require you to read the fine print.

California's religious exemption is more restrictive than many and is limited to groups that forbid seeking any medical care from traditional practitioners. Balancing this is the availability of philosophical exemption. That statute says, "Immunization of a person shall not be required" if the parent or guardian "files with the governing authority a letter or affidavit that documents which immunizations required have not been given on the basis that they are contrary to his or her beliefs." That sounds simple enough, but the state added a proviso in 2014 that parents must first be given "information regarding the benefits and risks of the immunization and the health risks of the communicable diseases" by an approved health care provider.

In other words, before you can opt out, you need to get a lecture from your health care professional. While annoying, this should not be a bar to getting the exemption. Our advice is not to get into a disagreement; just politely repeat your philosophical objection without elaboration, get the note, and go on your way.

Further undercutting parental choice, a law went into effect in California in 2013 that allows any child twelve or over to receive a vaccine against sexually transmitted diseases without parental consent. That means a young teen could receive the HPV vaccine during some kind of doctor's visit, based on their supposed need to protect themselves from sexually transmitted diseases based on their (possible) intention to become sexually active. If a vaccine reaction occurred, the parents would not necessarily suspect the cause. That's dangerous to the child, who probably would not want to acknowledge they had secretly gotten a vaccine linked to sexual activity.

So who, really, is putting children's well-being at risk here—careful parents or vaccine zealots?

In states that only allow religious beliefs as a basis for opting out, the bar can be much higher than for philosophical exemptions. To look again at our respective home states, Virginia and Massachusetts: Neither has philosophical exemptions, so unless your child has a recognized medical problem that would contraindicate vaccination, such as an immune deficiency caused by a genetic disorder or treatment such as chemotherapy, you will find yourself dealing with the tricky area of religious beliefs.

The Virginia form is short and simple: "The administration of immunizing agents conflicts with the above named student's/my religious tenets or practices. I understand, that in the occurrence of an outbreak, potential epidemic or epidemic of a vaccine-preventable disease in my/my child's school, the State Health Commissioner may order my/my child's exclusion from school, for my/my child's own protection, until the danger has passed." Sign the form in the presence of a notary public, and you are set.

In Massachusetts, information on medical and religious exemptions is combined on one form. Most of the material describes how unimmunized children can be banned from school during epidemics of measles, mumps, rubella, and so on. Regarding religious exemptions, it says merely: "a religious exemption is allowed if a parent or guardian submits a written statement that immunizations conflict with their sincere religious beliefs."

Given the ferocity with which vaccine advocates claim all children *must* be vaccinated, these are surprisingly mild requirements for claiming religious beliefs as a reason to be exempt. There's no requirement to say which religion or to prove membership in an organized or recognized group.

So once again the reality is not quite as ominous as you might expect. Just as states don't require for school attendance all vaccines recommended by the federal government—or agree on which ones to give—the opt-out, whether philosophical or even religious, is not always onerous.

At least in theory, that is. As parent concerns about the bloated and ever-increasing vaccine schedule have led to decreasing vaccination rates, public health officials have tried to crack down on such relatively easy outs.

New York State has led the way in trying to restrict the religious exemption. The wording itself is more threatening than in Virginia or Massachusetts:

"A religious exemption is a written and signed statement from the parent, parents or guardian of such child, stating that the parent, parents or guardian objects to their child's immunization due to sincere and genuine religious beliefs which prohibit the immunization of their child. The principal or person in charge of the school may require supporting documents. The *school decides* [emphasis added] whether to accept or reject the request for a religious exemption."

Not content with that, officials in some states have gone after parents with a vengeance. In a federal court case ostensibly focused on whether a court can bar unimmunized students from school during an epidemic, a Brooklyn-based judge said the U.S. Supreme Court has "strongly suggested that religious objectors are not constitutionally exempt from vaccinations."

As the *New York Times* reported, the judge "cited a 1905 Supreme Court ruling that upheld a $5 fine for a Massachusetts man who disobeyed an order to be vaccinated during a smallpox outbreak, a case that helped establish the government's right to require immunizations as a matter of public health."

One of the three families that brought the suit had been turned down for a religious exemption after the mother wrote: "I am requesting this religious exemption because it is my strong belief that all vaccines are made with toxic chemicals that are injected into the bloodstream by vaccination. According to the FDA all vaccines are made with foreign proteins (viruses & bacteria's), and some vaccines are even made with genetically engineered viral and bacterial materials. . . . I believe that man is made in God's image and the injection of toxic chemicals and foreign proteins into the bloodstream is a violation of God's directive to keep the body, (which is to be treated as a temple), holy and free from impurities . . ." Although not specifically ruling in her case, the court rejected her argument, saying it was not sufficiently grounded in religious reasoning.

Parents and vaccine-safety advocates will need to be vigilant and support each other as public health officials try to meet their caution with coercion. In 2012, Vermont legislators turned back an attempt to remove the philosophical exemption. They did add language similar to California's requiring parents who want to opt out to be informed about the risks to their children and others.

"Parents from the Vermont Coalition for Vaccine Choice blitzed legislators with emails, phone calls and conversations in the

Statehouse hallways," reported the *Burlington Free Press*. Said one pro-exemption parent, "The most dangerous place in the woods is between a mother bear and her cubs." Groups fighting for the parental right to make family-health choices are active in many states.

As we've said throughout this book, free speech and free choice tend to support each other, and efforts to silence vaccine concerns and curtail vaccine exemptions tend to go hand in hand. In 2010, we were invited to appear on New York's public radio station, WNYC, to speak about our book, *The Age of Autism*. The respected host, Leonard Lopate, told us on air: "Well, when we announced we were going to have you people on the show we were contacted by the New York City Department of Health and Mental Hygiene concerned that we were suggesting a link between mercury and autism. You must have known you were stirring up a hornet's nest when you wrote this book. Are you prepared for all the attacks that are sure to follow?

"Oh, we get attacked on a pretty regular basis," Mark Blaxill responded. "We've become accustomed to that. I think one of the things that we really need to recover in this whole debate is a sense of civil discourse, and an ability to take on controversial subjects in an open-minded way."

Some parents seeking exemptions as a way out of vaccine mandates have turned to relatively new and unorthodox solutions—like joining the Universal Family Church, founded in 2010, which asserts among its tenets that "decisions made by fathers and mothers regarding the best course of action for their children's spiritual and physical health should be honored in almost all situations. We believe no government or other authority has a greater right to determine what is best for your family."

Universal Family Church (UFC) is a multi-faith church, in some respects modeled on The Society For Ethical Culture, a recognized religion founded in 1876. Like the Society, UFC members can retain their own religious affiliation: "We believe regardless of your religious affiliation that you can obtain a relationship with God whether your core faith is Buddhism, Christianity, Hinduism, Islam and Judaism, etc."

Some families have been able to obtain religious exemptions by joining this organization and citing it as the basis of their beliefs.

Facing the Pressure to Conform

Just because we are outlining logical steps based on your legal right to vaccine choice, we don't suggest this is an easy or cut-and-dried path. At any point along the way you can encounter resistance, ranging from a tut-tut at a playgroup followed by no more invitations to play dates, to being kicked out of a longtime family doctor's practice, to being barred from school, to being confronted in an emergency room by a doctor demanding you vaccinate *right now,* to a visit from child protective services enquiring about all aspects of your home life with your child's vaccine status as a wedge issue.

What we do argue is that just like everything else that's important in life, you must prevail in defending your right to keep your child healthy. You must stand up for yourself, your family, and the fundamental American right to choose what you put in your baby's body. If you do, as we said in the first section, you will find you're not alone.

If you don't, and problems occur, you'll find yourself very alone indeed. Listen to the voices of some parents of vaccine-damaged children on Facebook, asked what they wish they'd known and would have done differently:

- I wish I had understood that vaccine reactions are cumulative. Reactions like fever, rash, swelling, lethargy, sleeping for days, are cumulative and add up to autism. They are all reactions and an assault to the immune system. At 2 months [my son] screamed inconsolably after a round of 8 vaccines. That was his brain swelling. Doctor said it was "normal". I wish I had listened to my inner voice that said, "don't do it." I wish I had investigated each ingredient in every vaccine given to my child. I wish I had not given him Tylenol or antibiotics.
- I would do so many things differently. The first thing would be to listen to that mother's instinct and actually act on it. I would have learned more about the mainstream prenatal and birthing process and also looked at natural/home birth

options and/or hired a doula or midwife. As far as vaccines, I would have read more about the body's immune system, the diseases vaccines are supposedly reducing, and then really read up on vaccines, their ingredients and the reactions that can happen. Diet is another thing I would have looked at and taken more seriously. So many things factor in our health and the choices we make.

- I wish I had followed my instincts to not vaccinate. I saw my son suffer a reaction to the DTaP right before my eyes. I would not have been induced either. We have practically lost the roof over our heads trying to provide therapies, education and treatment because insurance would not cover anything. This whole experience has been a nightmare and the worst of it is watching our child suffer discrimination by the teachers and a city school system so callous it deliberately disregards children's educational needs and fights parents tooth and nail against obtaining even 1:1 ABA (Applied Behavior Analysis therapy). I don't wish this on any child or parent. Seeing how my child gets treated through the process is agonizing. Avoid vaccines.

The consistent theme is regret at not following a parent's instincts. This is why no one path is right for every parent, because each must listen to his or her own inner voice. But it all begins and ends at the same point: Having enough confidence, conviction, and, yes, courage, to educate yourself and refuse to abdicate personal choice on behalf of your child.

CHAPTER 16

HOW TO PREVENT VACCINE INJURIES

IF YOU CHOOSE TO VACCINATE, there are a number of ways to minimize risk, along with adopting an alternative schedule. Here is a compendium of ideas to consider.

- Don't get any shots before two months of age. No vaccine was recommended at such an early age until the hep B shot at birth in 1991. A baby's immune system has not even begun developing when it emerges from the birth canal. It's dangerous to interfere with something so fragile so quickly.
- Don't get any shot containing ethylmercury (still in many flu shots). Read the label, and if you see the word thimerosal—ethylmercury—run.
- Don't get any vaccines during pregnancy. The CDC now advises all pregnant women to get a flu shot and a Tdap shot.
- Don't have elective dental work during or shortly before pregnancy, and don't have dental amalgams removed during that period. Mercury vapor can move easily through the body and get to the fetus quickly.
- Don't let your baby get more than two injections at one time. Elizabeth Mumper follows that strategy, giving one shot in each thigh. If a reaction occurs, the doctor and parent can narrow it down quickly and perhaps change strategy if a booster is due.
- Limit the problem of viral interference, actually getting sick as a result of being exposed to multiple viruses at the same time,

by getting only one live-virus shot per visit. At the same twelve-month, well-baby checkup, an infant could get MMR and chicken pox shots containing live viruses, thereby requiring your baby's immune system to develop its protections against all of them at the same time. Postpone the MMR and chicken pox vaccines, and put at least a month between them. Viral interference is too big a risk to do otherwise.

- If you believe your child was injured by a vaccine or were concerned by a reaction, stop vaccinating as usual. If that child has younger siblings, stop vaccinating them or proceed with extreme caution. Siblings of children with autism have a much higher risk of developing the disorder, perhaps because of a shared genetic vulnerability, such as inability to detoxify properly, or an underlying mitochondrial anomaly or environmental exposure.

- Do breastfeed if possible, for a year at minimum. Dr. Mayer Eisenstein at Homefirst said that in his children, "we have virtually no asthma if you're breast-fed and not vaccinated."

- Avoid commercial dairy products, especially milk, after weaning. Mumper said she has been able to disrupt the common cycle of ear infections and antibiotics by switching children away from dairy. That also reduces the rationale for the pneumococcal vaccine, which is believed to cut down on ear infections.

- Don't vaccinate a baby that's sick or on antibiotics, or has been recently. Anything that disrupts the natural balance of gut bacteria can throw off the immune system in dangerous ways.

- Do consider products that promote the development of your baby's least developed organs: probiotics, Vitamin D, and Vitamin A, which encourage healthy immune and gut function.

- Eat organic foods and avoid pesticide exposure in any other way you can. Several studies have linked pesticide exposure to autism, asthma, and ADHD, as well as adult-neurological diseases like Parkinson's. The link makes sense—anything that disrupts brain function in one species (insects) might do so in another (humans). Our own research brought this home: We've proposed that polio was a benign virus until the advent of modern pesticides—starting with lead arsenate in the 1890s and continuing through the DDT era—allowed the virus to gain access to the nervous system where it became far more dangerous and even fatal. A number of other "mystery diseases" afflicting children—from an outbreak of tics in rural New York high schools to baffling paralysis among children in California—may have their roots in pesticides and other commercial toxins, we believe. Avoid them.

- Likewise, try not to live downwind of coal plants or near Superfund sites or other reservoirs and emitters of toxins. All have been associated with a higher risk of autism and other disorders. We believe the rise of pollution from the Industrial Revolution triggered a host of previously unheard-of diseases, including schizophrenia, a topic we discuss at length in our first book.

- Avoid toxins in the house and surroundings. Don't use products like flea-killing pet shampoos while pregnant; one disturbing study linked them to a higher rate of autism. Likewise, don't undertake major home remodeling or landscaping during or around pregnancy. We've talked to a number of parents who believe such exposures contributed to their child's disorder.

- If you use day care—55 percent of Americans do—look for a setting that's as small as possible. Mumper says that groups of half a dozen or fewer kids seem to pose less risk for respiratory illness or diarrhea.

- Don't take acetaminophen to prevent or treat fever from vaccination. Many vaccine-safety advocates believe acetaminophen inhibits the liver's ability to detoxify, and a number of scientific studies support that view.

- Be aware of autoimmunity issues in your family. From the first reports of autism in 1943, family predisposition to autoimmune disorders has flashed a bright-red warning, one that the medical community has been tragically slow to see. Thyroid issues in the mother seem particularly problematic, but eczema, asthma, lupus, and similar disorders in either parent, in siblings, or in collateral relations, should be taken seriously.

- Read the Vaccine Information Statement provided by the CDC as it relates to side effects. Also take the time to Google and read the vaccine's official product label provided by the manufacturer, a lengthier and scarier document. Remember this when you see the word "encephalopathy": It means brain damage, and brain damage can result in ADHD, seizures, and the behavioral syndrome that characterizes "autism." There is substantial evidence from government concessions in the Vaccine Injury Compensation Program that autism is a common outcome of the vaccine injury labeled "encephalopathy."
- A good resource is MAPS (www.medmaps.org), an organization of doctors who treat special-needs kids. MAPS is also plugged into other medical providers who take a whole-body approach to wellness and disease prevention.

Our friend Sylvia Pimentel provides an eloquent summary as she describes her two sons with autism, both of whom she believes were cases of vaccine injury:

Our oldest son Joseph regressed after several vaccine appointments. Yes, the obscenely ironically named Well-Baby appointments. But we had no idea regression was even possible from vaccines. We kept thinking that he caught some sort of bug or virus at the doctor's office, and was sick, so that was why he was screaming and had such bad diarrhea. And when he lost eye contact and couldn't communicate any more, we thought it was because he wasn't recovered from his illness yet. But about the time we realized he was behind developmentally, I was about to give birth to our youngest son, Nicholas. So I was determined to do everything by the book with him. With Joseph, I had never given him Tylenol with his vaccines, even though that is what the doctor advised us to do. I just didn't feel comfortable giving drugs that weren't needed. (Yes, I now understand the irony of that statement since we were allowing him to be injected with dozens of unneeded vaccines. . . .)

With Nick, I was determined to do everything "by the book," so I obediently followed all doctor orders, which included giving Nick Tylenol before and after vaccine appointments. But Nick's reactions after each set of shots were ten times worse than Joseph's ever were. *Profoundly* high-pitched screaming with arched back, which I now know is a key sign of brain swelling. Severe projectile vomiting. Fever. Profuse, explosive diarrhea. Repeated calls to the pediatricians led nowhere. I was told that "most babies are fussy after vaccines" and to give "more Tylenol." Well, that was the absolute *worst* thing we could have done. You see, Tylenol depletes glutathione, and the body needs glutathione to detoxify poisons—such as the poisons that are in vaccines. And it turns out some years later we did a bunch of testing on Nick, and he is missing one of the genes that produce glutathione. So destroying what little he had was like pouring grease on a fire.

So: by giving Nicholas Tylenol while vaccinating him, he is much more severely autistic than his older brother.

Vaccines are dangerous. Giving Tylenol with vaccines, which to this very day is standard practice, is insanely, recklessly dangerous.

If Something Goes Wrong

Vaccine reactions are unpredictable, but they are very real. Some are immediate and life threatening, others delayed and chronic. Especially because the medical practice that administered the vaccine may be loath to acknowledge any problems, it is important to know what adverse events to watch for; how to treat, document, and report them, and, if necessary, seek compensation. We hope this never happens to you or your family—that's why we've written this book! We believe that being a careful medical consumer greatly reduces the chances.

Let's start with one of the worst, but by no means rare, symptoms—the one described by Sylvia Pimentel. Sharp, high-pitched screaming after vaccination, sometimes accompanied by an arched back and continuing for hours, is a deeply worrisome sign. Don't let anyone tell you it is just "screaming baby syndrome" (as a pediatrician told a friend of ours, whose infant went on to have seizures after another vaccination) or just a coincidence when it closely follows vaccination.

Screaming indicates swelling in the brain—encephalitis. And it needs prompt attention.

Febrile seizures from vaccination are treated by medical professionals as scary but ultimately harmless. But again, we believe they can be signs of possible permanent damage—especially fevers well above 100 degrees that persist for several days. Make sure you see your health care provider and insist on your belief that a vaccination is the likely trigger.

In one case, in which a child named Bailey Banks was compensated by the VICP for MMR vaccine injury that led to an autistic disorder, the parents had demanded that the child receive a brain scan immediately. It captured inflammation that might have been missed just a few days later.

With the advent of cell-phone video recorders, anyone can document problems after vaccination. Most parents need no invitation to do so, but we suggest you record your child's milestones—birth, one month, three months, six months, and so on—and also immediately before well-baby visits that may include vaccination. Studies have proven that autistic regression does occur, and if you have the video, you'll be in a much better position to seek redress.

We're creating a smartphone app that can walk you through this process and the following steps.

If you think your child has suffered a vaccine injury, you should report it to your doctor and ask them to file a report with the Vaccine Adverse Events Reporting System (VAERS). Also, file one yourself; the system is voluntary and your health care provider may choose not to file. Even if your provider dismisses your concern and won't file, parents are allowed to file on their own.

You can also file a request for compensation with the Vaccine Injury Compensation Program. Unfortunately, this is the vaccine "court" that is implicitly condoning the rise of vaccine injury through its fundamentally flawed procedures and mistreatment of injured parties. This bureaucracy helps perpetuate the myths by dismissing vaccine injury as coincidence and promoting a false sense of security regarding vaccine safety. It has already tossed out more than 5,000 autism claims brought under an "omnibus" action and continually shortened the list of "table injuries" following within a prescribed time after vaccination that automatically trigger a successful claim.

Nonetheless, the court, financed by a 75 cent tax paid by consumers on every vaccine, has paid out more than $2.8 billion, demonstrating both the reality of severe vaccine injury and the fact that, at least in some cases, justice is done.

CHAPTER 17

THE FUTURE OF HEALTHY KIDS

THE WAY WE JUDGE THE SUCCESS OF medical interventions should be total-health outcomes.

But what if everyone adopts an alternative approach or no vaccines at all? In other words, would the success of the model we're advocating lead to consequences that raise serious questions about whether it's a good idea? When Barack Obama was asked about vaccine choice by the mother of a vaccine-injured child during his first presidential race, he said, "I believe that it will bring back deadly diseases, like polio."

Fortunately, that is not the choice we really face. The United States has by far the most aggressive vaccine schedule in the world, but far from the healthiest kids. Sweden ranks at the top of that list, with an infant-mortality rate less than half that of the United States.

And its vaccine schedule, while protecting against the same serious diseases, is much different.

- *No* universal hep B vaccine (recommended only for children at risk, with hep B-positive mothers)
- *No* rotavirus vaccine
- *No* influenza vaccine
- *No* hep A vaccine
- *No* meningococcal vaccine

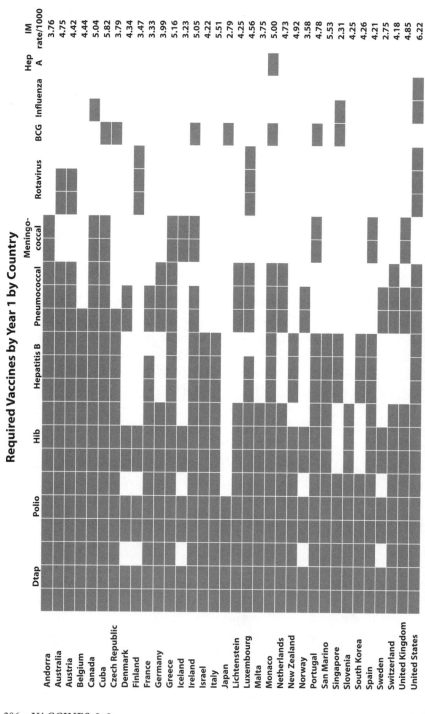

Required Vaccines by Year 1 by Country

- *No* chicken pox vaccine—these first six vaccines constitute much of the bloat we're talking about when we refer to the "bloated" US vaccination schedule.
- Three diphtheria, Hib, and pneumococcal shots in infancy, not four; all starting at three months, not two.
- Three polio shots in infancy starting at three months, not two months.
- The MMR vaccine at eighteen months, not twelve.
- Gardasil®, for girls only, at twelve to thirteen years, not eleven to twelve.

In almost every way, Sweden and most other developed countries appear more cautious and more delayed in their vaccine schedules. And their children are healthier.

The real choice, then, is between chronic and developmental conditions that are ignored in a quixotic hunt for a disease-free world, versus one that balances the threat of deadly diseases against the new disorders increasingly crippling us in an entirely different way. We don't believe in wars—against disease, against vaccination, or otherwise. We *do* believe in balance, safety, and caution.

As we finished this book, we reached out to Anthony M., the Concerned Father we quoted at the start whose New Year's baby, London, prompted him to ask about reliable vaccine information. "Were you able to come up with an approach you feel comfortable with and the doctors accepted?" we asked. "And how is your beautiful baby girl getting along?"

He responded that she is unvaccinated, "much to the chagrin of the doctor" who saw her the one time she was ill. He continued:

> Honestly my wife and I remain bewildered at how the powers that be attempt to "execute" mandatory shots. But we both maintain a healthy suspicion of the process, and if we can hold out and send her to private schooling then that's what it will be. Of course anytime I see other kids who have been vaccinated and appear fine I can't help but wonder if we're

doing the right thing. Yet the fact remains that my wife and I could not in good conscience introduce foreign elements into her body if we are not fully convinced of their safety (not to mention purpose).

He included a picture of his bright-eyed daughter, looking and pointing directly at the camera—signs she's meeting key developmental milestones. Clearly, this family's choice will not be everyone's. But we hope everyone finds the same health and happiness along whatever path they choose.

ACKNOWLEDGEMENTS

Writers don't exist without readers, and our first thanks go to them:

Readers of our blog, AgeOfAutism.com, whose comments and conversations are reflected, directly or indirectly, in these pages.

Readers of our first book —*The Age of Autism: Mercury, Medicine, and a Man-made Epidemic*—where we set out ideas that led to this one.

Early readers of *Vaccines 2.0*: Jennifer Larson, who helped us come up with the book and its focus; Katie Weisman, Ginger Taylor, and Kim Mack Rosenberg, who offered valuable advice; Gayle DeLong, who shared her groundbreaking analysis of vaccine-injury data; and Laura Hayes, who made us think hard about what we wanted to say.

Our colleagues at Age Of Autism, at HealthChoice, and at the Canary Party deserve our special thanks.

shots

References and citations can be found at
www.skyhorsepublishing.com

Quotes from Internet sources such as blog comments and
comment threads have been left as they originally appeared.
Such quotes may include spelling, grammatical, and
typographical errors.